Handling the Handicapped

Handling the Handicapped

A guide to the lifting
and movement of disabled people

springer publishing company, inc.

200 Park Avenue South • New York, New York 10003

Woodhead-Faulkner Ltd
7 Rose Crescent
Cambridge CB2 3LL

First published 1975
Second impression 1976
Third impression 1977

©

The Chartered Society of Physiotherapy
1975

ISBN 0 85941 012 9 (Paper)
ISBN 0 85941 063 3 (Cased)

Printed in Great Britain by
The Burlington Press
Foxton, Royston, Herts.

FOREWORD

The Baroness Masham of Ilton

At the outset I should like to thank the Chartered Society of Physiotherapy for offering me the privilege of contributing a Foreword to this much-needed book. I am sure that the information it contains, which is written by experts, will be of benefit to many people.

The book has been published primarily to show the correct manner in which handicapped people should be lifted and moved, and as such will be of help to all those—whether relatives, friends, physiotherapists, nurses or members of voluntary organisations—who live or work with the handicapped. If one is not aware of the proper procedures to be followed, it is very easy to cause permanent damage to oneself by lifting a handicapped person the wrong way.

Handicapped people themselves will also derive great relief from knowing that those around them are being educated to their needs. As Chairman of the newly formed Spinal Injuries Association and a paraplegic myself, I know only too well the many problems which severely handicapped people and their families have to overcome. The greatest wish of the handicapped is to be able to live in the community as independently as possible, but being lifted is one of the most essential parts of their daily living.

Great numbers of handicapped people are elderly, suffering from the results of rheumatic and arthritic complaints. If a great deal of pain is to be avoided, skilled handling is essential and the book rightly stresses the need for thorough assessment.

I therefore commend this book to all those who are concerned with caring for the handicapped and hope that it will succeed in attracting a wide readership.

ACKNOWLEDGEMENTS

The authors of Chapters 3, 4, 7 and 8 would like to acknowledge the co-operation they received from the staff, patients and voluntary helpers at Winford Orthopaedic Hospital, Bristol, and Bierley Hall Hospital, Bradford, during the taking of the photographs that illustrate these chapters.

The voluntary helpers had to learn the lifts in order to be photographed. Their energy was unflagging and their willingness to learn was a great source of inspiration to the authors.

CONTENTS

Chapter 1

INTRODUCTION

J. Henry Smith, B.E.M., M.C.S.P., Dip.T.P.

A handicapped person suffers from psychological as well as physical disadvantages. He has to rely to a great extent on other people to help him to move about, and he feels defenceless and at the mercy of those who handle his body—not only hospital staff but also family, friends and helpers. The approach of someone who is handling a handicapped person is therefore all-important: it can make or mar the relationship between them.

The human hand, which is a unique instrument of communication, has a profound influence in establishing *rapport* between the handicapped person and the handler. By its touch it can comfort and reassure, and stimulate physical response and reflex action. For those people, such as physiotherapists, who are skilled in examining patients by use of their hands, the hand feeds back a wealth of information which will influence subsequent handling and treatment. Applied carelessly or incorrectly, the hand will, however, arouse hostility, which finds expression in unfavourable muscular and emotional reactions. It then becomes difficult for the handler to gain the active co-operation of the person being handled —particularly if his or her functional abilities are seriously impaired.

Good handling depends on using, as far as practicable, the whole palm of the hand. This provides a secure but comfortable hold which both allows the handler to control the part of the body to be moved or stabilised, and gives confidence to the person being handled. The handler should always avoid gripping with the finger ends. This leads to the use of needless force, does not provide a really secure hold, and through localised pressure may cause discomfort to the patient and inhibit his co-operation.

In making contact with any part of the body which is to be moved, the handler should move his fully opened hand smoothly and gently in the direction required by the subsequent manoeuvre. This will supply the correct initial stimulus. When a limb is to be moved, it should be lifted, supported and carried from below. This

1

"carrying" action is an essential feature of good handling, and follows naturally from efficient use by the handler of her own body.

Handling the handicapped demands considerable physical effort, and there will be far less risk of strain if the handler cultivates skill rather than the use of strength. But, however skilful the handler may become, she must recognise her limitations, and never undertake on her own a task which requires the combined efforts of several people.

Wherever possible, the handler should use the handicapped person's weight to advantage. Changing the position of a limb or limbs will also change the distribution of weight, and this can greatly assist certain movements, such as turning over in bed. The efficiency and ease with which any action is performed depends on how it is initiated. In lifting, for example, the position of the lifter's body is not the only criterion: it is the *condition* of the body resulting from the way it *moves into position* which is significant. In other words, the lifter must prepare her own body to carry out the lift. Thus, lowering the hands in preparation for a lift should be brought about by first relaxing the knees while at the same time keeping the trunk upright and the head erect. By lowering the body base in this way one avoids the top-heavy unbalanced movement resulting from bending forward from the waist—a common source of back strain. Although relaxing at the knees is in effect bending the knees, thinking in terms of relaxation encourages an easy, rhythmic type of movement which should start before the load is taken and then follow through into the final stages of lifting and lowering.

Furthermore, when the handler moves into action, as just described, the feet will readily assume a good position to enable the body to remain in balance when the load is taken and to provide effective thrust for the lift. The body must be well balanced at all stages, and this depends on proper positioning of the feet. In general, this means the feet should be reasonably apart, with one foot forward and pointing in the direction of movement.

The handler initiates the actual lift by raising the crown of her head and gently tucking in her chin. This helps to stabilise the spinal column, and reduces the danger of straining the back and shoulders. Force for the lift is derived from the powerful leg muscles, which must continue to operate smoothly and rhythmically throughout the transfer and lowering of the load.

Good movement and handling techniques cannot be learned only from a book: the reader must also practise and experiment with able-bodied people to make sure she knows what she is doing, before she attempts to handle a handicapped person. As with so many other things, practice makes perfect.

Having to depend on others for your daily needs can mean a loss of dignity and self-respect, but it can go a long way to restoring them if the handicapped person is made to feel that he has a contribution to make—no matter how small—to the joint enterprise of dealing with his problems.

Handling the handicapped involves a close personal relationship between helpers and the person being dealt with; efficient handling requires firm physical contact, and this must be mutually recognised and accepted from the outset. A tentative or uncertain approach will undermine confidence, and make any manoeuvre more difficult and less effective.

There are many sick and disabled persons in whom pain will have the last word when they are being handled: it will determine how much physical help the patient will be able to give, and how much handling he will be able to tolerate. Pain varies greatly not just from day to day but from hour to hour. The handler has to depend entirely on the patient for guidance, and must keep asking him if the hold being used is painful, so that he is not forced beyond his tolerance. In some situations certainly discomfort and some degree of pain is unavoidable, but it must always be kept to the practical minimum.

The value of first assessing the problem, and then planning and organising to deal with it, cannot be over-emphasised. Time spent on this at the start will save much time later on, avoid wasted effort and spare frayed tempers. Each situation should be assessed individually (as described in Chapter 2), and a co-ordinated plan laid down in which the handicapped person should participate to the extent of his physical and mental capacity. This will boost his morale and make him feel he is a member of the team.

Team spirit, indeed, is an essential factor in handling the handicapped when more than one helper is involved. One person should act as leader--of the team, and should decide—after listening to any suggestions the handicapped person may have—what is the best method to employ. The leader should make her intentions quite clear to the person to be lifted and to the other helpers, so that when she gives an agreed signal the operation can be carried out with smoothness and precision. Good-humoured systematic working along these lines helps to remove any impression of haste. However pressing other matters may be, it is essential to avoid any suggestion of impatience: many handicapped people are very sensitive about the demands they make on the time of those who help them.

Comfortable clothing is important also, both for the helpers and for the handicapped person; the latter should wear clothes permitting free movement without undue exposure, which will help to preserve dignity and conserve body heat. Helpers should wear clothes which do not restrict their movement, and make for ease in handling; sensible footwear, too, is essential for safety.

The fundamental principles of handling and lifting as described in this introduction always remain constant, but their application must vary for each occasion. The one criterion that must always be observed is to use common sense and humanity.

Chapter 2

ASSESSING THE SITUATION

S. Y. Saywell, F.C.S.P.

Before you start to handle a handicapped person, it is essential first to assess the situation, and then to plan and organise what you are going to do. Every situation, and every patient, will be different, and so a separate assessment must be made each time.

Aims of Assessment

There are three aims to bear in mind when you are making your assessment:

1. Try to find out what limitations the handicapped person has because of his disability, and also what his capabilities are: in other words, what he can and can't do.

2. Help yourself to overcome your own natural fear as a layman, by finding out exactly what you will have to do in each individual situation, by familiarising yourself with different types of handicap so that you do not recoil from them, and by having a known task to perform among strangers in an unfamiliar setting.

3. Give the handicapped person confidence in you as someone who is experienced and appreciates his difficulties.

You will make it much easier for yourself if you remember always to think of the handicapped person as an individual who is unfortunate enough to have a disability and who requires your help, instead of concentrating on the problem and forgetting the person involved.

Sight, Speech and Hearing

It is important to find out if the handicapped person's sight, speech and hearing are defective in any way. This is done by questioning him and noting how he responds to simple commands. His response will also reveal something of his personality—whether he is happy or morose, timid or courageous, whether he is eager to please, or seeks attention. You will begin to find out whether he has an independent nature, or has to lean on others, and how able he is to cope with the frustrations of his handicap.

How to Make Your Assessment

Let us assume that the handicapped person is in a wheelchair. First you will find out his name and age, and what is wrong with him.

1. To test his hand and arm control, greet him by name and shake hands with him. This will give you an idea of how strong his grip is. Comment on this, and ask him to grip you with his other hand, so that you may compare the two. While you are doing this you should note the action of his hands and arms, seeing whether it is normal or unusual in any way. You should also note the firmness of his grasp, and whether he is able to release it easily or not. Another thing to look for is how much movement he uses in order to make contact with you: that is to say, whether he is limited to wrist movements or can move his arms from the elbow or shoulder; whether he leans his whole trunk forward, and perhaps moves his neck as well.

2. Observe his head and neck closely, to find out if he has normal control of them or if there is too much movement, and if he can follow movement in others by turning his head and neck or can only use his eyes.

3. Next you should test the handicapped person's control of his trunk movements by asking him to lean forward, and then to sit upright again. Note whether he does this easily, or is stiff and rigid in his movement, or his movement is uncontrolled and he bends or falls forward. He may also be unable to regain his upright position. Then you should ask him to turn his trunk from side to side, and to bend it from side to side, so that you see in each case whether he does this easily or with some difficulty.

4. Control of the arms must next be tested and this is done by asking the handicapped person:

    (a) To raise both arms forward at shoulder level.
    (b) To raise both arms above his head.

(c) To raise both arms sideways.

(d) To put his right hand behind his head and his left behind his back, and try to join the fingers of both hands. He should then be asked to do this with the arms in the reverse positions.

Observe his movements carefully, so that you know exactly what his capabilities are.

5. The legs are tested in much the same way, by asking the patient:

(a) To stretch each leg forward from the knee, and then bend it back again.

(b) To lift each leg independently from the hip, and return it to its former position.

(c) To work each foot up and down.

(d) To circle each foot.

Note the speed and strength of each movement, and whether it is performed with ease or difficulty.

6. Lastly, you test the handicapped person's ability to stand, balance and walk. Ask him to stand up from his wheelchair, and note if he needs any help to do this. Then ask him to take a few steps forward, and see if he needs support or not. Ask him to stand on one leg and to raise the other as though mounting a step, and check whether or not he can take his weight on the standing leg. Finally, ask him to turn in a small circle, and to sit down, noting once again any difficulties he may have.

All this testing takes very little time, but reveals to the helper the extent of the problem. For instance, can it be coped with single-handed, or will help be needed? If the latter, will one or more extra helpers be required? Will any sort of mechanical aid or hoist be necessary? How much is the handicapped person able to contribute to the operation himself?

Some Common Difficulties

1. The handicapped person may be top-heavy, which will present the lifters with a problem of balance. His trunk will require

more support, and you must be careful not to lift his legs, or he will overbalance.

2. If the handicapped person is reasonably independent, the speed of movement of the lift must be controlled by his capabilities —not yours.

3. If two or more handlers are working together as a team, don't forget that one must be the leader, and that all must work together when the leader gives a pre-arranged signal.

4. Deaf or mentally subnormal people will present a problem. It is important to hold their attention all the time you are working with them.

5. Blind or partially blind people must have an oral explanation of everything you propose to do. Don't forget that they cannot see you, or that you may be just a dim shape. Introduce yourself and any other helpers, and explain every move clearly and comprehensively.

Know Your Own Limitations

It is most important to be able to recognise a situation where you will need professional help. One example is when the handicapped person has a sudden spasm in a limb, which might throw a helper off balance. Another example is when the legs are rigid, and cannot be separated or bent.

In such cases don't be afraid to acknowledge that the situation is beyond your own capabilities, and to ask for professional help.

Chapter 3

RULES AND MECHANICAL PRINCIPLES

P. J. Waddington, M.C.S.P., Dip.T.P.
M. Hollis, M.B.E., M.C.S.P., Dip.T.P.

Introduction

When a handicapped person is being moved from one place or position to another, it is important that the helper and the handicapped should move together as one, and that there should be one or more fixed points around which the load pivots. (The exception is when several people are working together to lift someone completely clear of the ground.) If a partially handicapped person is moving himself, he can keep his feet, hands, buttocks or head in a fixed position to act as a pivot. If a helper is moving a handicapped person, she will usually immobilise, or "fix", his feet and possibly also his knees. To do this she stands obliquely to him and, if his feet are on the floor, she blocks the toe of his shoe with her instep and his knee with the inside of her knee. Both the handicapped person and the helper should wear firmly fitting shoes, for safety. In this position the helper's feet are also fixed, and the feet of both will form one joint fixed point to act as a pivot about which both can move in unison.

Unless a handicapped person is properly held in the erect position, his body may easily "crumple". In order to hold him erect, his knees, sacrum (the bony area above the buttocks) and shoulders may be used as "locking points" (Fig. 1). If the helper applies properly balanced pressure at these points, the handicapped person will be held upright until he feels balanced and ready to control his erect posture by himself. The helper can support the handicapped person and forestall any tendencies of his body to lean by using close contact with her own body. Thus, if he has a tendency to lean towards her, she pushes towards him, and, if he leans away, she pulls back. In other words, the two bodies support each other, and the helper helps the handicapped person to stay erect.

9

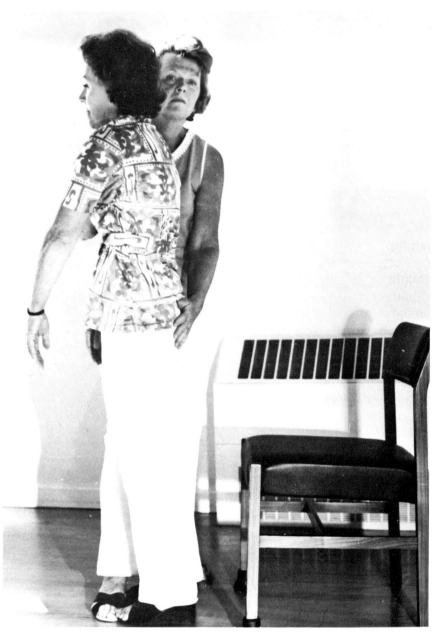

Fig. 1.   *The feet are "blocked", the knees, the bony area above the buttocks and the shoulders are "locked", and by counterpressures the handicapped person is held erect*

When people lose some degree of their strength, whether temporarily or permanently, they may have to make several attempts at making a movement before they achieve it. After each unsuccessful attempt they will use greater effort, until they succeed—just as on a garden swing one merely touches the ground with a foot to start the movement, and uses increasingly stronger movements of the body and legs to increase the arc of the swing. This swinging movement may be used to help a handicapped person, with carefully timed assistance from the helper. Timing is an important part of the skill of helping a handicapped person to achieve a movement with the minimum effort. The helper should be careful to keep her assistance in time with the motion of the part of the handicapped person's body which is moving: particularly when helping him to stand from the sitting position, or to move from a bed to a chair, for instance. The direction of lifting should never be straight up, or straight forward, but always oblique or in the line of natural movement. It is the head or the buttocks which usually initiate movement of the body. Thus, in standing up or sitting up or rolling over, the head should always be moved first—and the handicapped person should not forget to look where he is going. In sitting down or turning backward the buttocks lead the way, while the head often moves in the opposite direction.

Rocking backward and forward from the hips is a movement that occurs naturally in laughter or in grief, but it can also be used to initiate a movement of the body which is difficult for a handicapped person to achieve. The rocking movement will at first be small, but it can be increased by pushing with the hands or pulling on a nearby fixed object. With well-timed assistance from a helper, the rocking movement can be greater still, and a rotary or turning motion can be added.

Each hip can in turn be moved forward or backward by rocking sideways from one hip to the other, at the same time pushing or pulling with the hands, so that a handicapped person can move towards the edge of the chair on which he is sitting in order to transfer himself to another piece of furniture, such as a bed. The only means of achieving this sideways rocking movement with a person who is very handicapped may be for the helper to use alternate pressure on his shoulders. In order to move in this way to the edge of a chair without scraping the back of the thighs or pulling up clothing, when the weight is on one buttock the opposite leg should be lifted. More than one rocking movement may be needed before the other leg can be moved.

Basic Holds for Helpers

These are as follows:

1. Wrist grip.
2. Finger grip.
3. Through-arm lift grip.
4. Palm-to-palm thumb grasp.
5. Forearm grasp.
6. Pelvic holds (hips).
7. Armpit hold.
8. Elbow grip.
9. Holds for adjusting the handicapped person's position.

1. Wrist grip (Fig. 2)
When two helpers are working together to lift a handicapped person, this and the following hold will enable the helpers to take a secure grip of *each other.*

2. Finger grip (Fig. 3)

3. Through-arm lift grip
This hold may be used by either one or two helpers. When selecting this hold one helper should ensure that the handicapped person has some power in the shoulders, or at least in one arm and hand (Fig. 4) when the handicapped person grasps his own wrist.

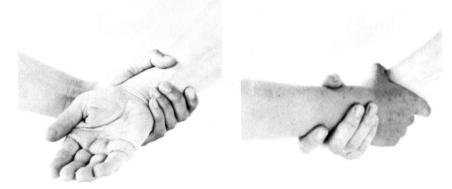

Fig. 2.   *The wrist grip.* Left: *the other hand is relaxed for support.* Right: *both helpers grip*

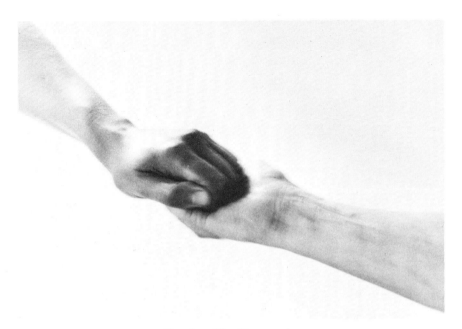

Fig. 3.   *The finger grip*

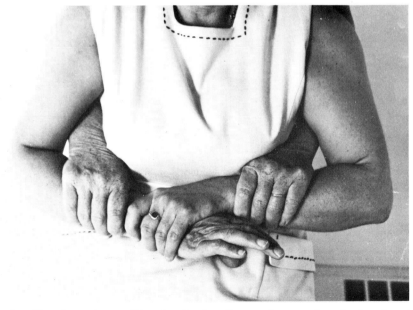

Fig. 4.   *The through-arm lift grip: the handicapped person's gripping hand must have enough power for this*

4. Palm-to-palm thumb grasp

This and the following holds are to be used when assisting a handicapped person to stand, transfer from one position to another, or walk.

The position of the helper's feet is astride with the front foot facing the direction of movement. The helper's second arm should be placed in one of three positions:

(a) So that her forearm is between the handicapped person's arm and chest wall near to but not in the armpit. On no account should the helper grip the upper arm as this will cause discomfort.

(b) Holding the elbow straight (Figs. 5 and 6).

(c) Round the waist.

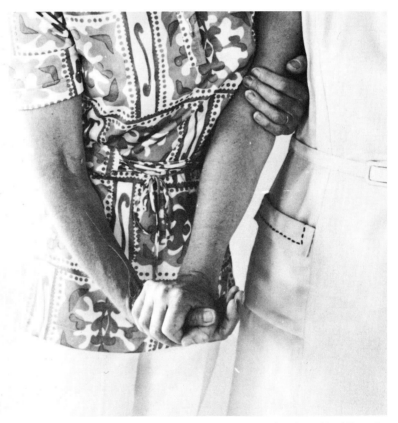

Fig. 5. *The palm-to-palm thumb grasp, showing the other hand holding the elbow straight*

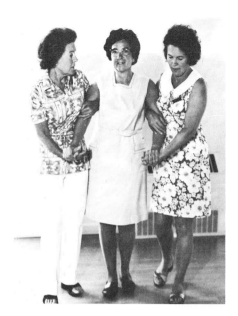

Fig. 6. *The palm-to-palm thumb grasp, showing the other hand holding the upper arm*

5. Forearm grasp

The handicapped person must have moderate power in both arms. This is used by one helper to assist the handicapped person from sitting to standing (Fig. 7). The helper stands in front with one foot in front, as in walking.

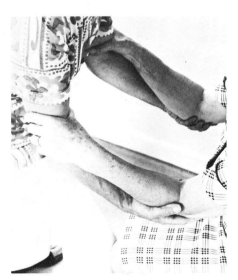

Fig. 7. *The forearm grasp: the helper's forearms are palm facing upwards under the handicapped person's elbows*

15

6. Pelvic holds (hips)

These are valuable for use with a more severely handicapped person. They give good control of the pelvis and hips. The helper stands facing the handicapped person, with one foot in front, as in walking. The forward leg may be positioned so that the helper's knee can "block" the handicapped person's knee. The hips and knees are bent and the back is straight. *There are three methods:*

(a) The helper's thumbs are inserted inside the waistband of the handicapped person's trousers or skirt, one on either side at the level of the seam. She grasps the garment with the whole hand.

(b) If the helper can reach, the hands may be placed palm up under the buttocks.

(c) In some cases, particularly with a weak heavy person, the pull on the trousers may cause discomfort in the crutch. Under these circumstances a belt around the waist may be used but this does not give good control of the pelvis and hips (Fig. 8).

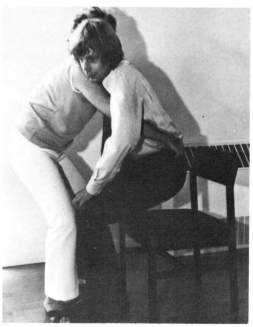

Fig. 8. *The pelvic hold using the waist-band: note the close contact and "blocking" position of the helper's legs*

7. Armpit hold

The helper stands as for the clothing hold (**6**(a) above) and puts the fingers, bent only at the knuckles, under the armpits. The fingers are inserted from the rear of the armpit on the side near the helper and from in front on the side furthest away, fingers turned palm upwards as much as possible (Fig. 9).

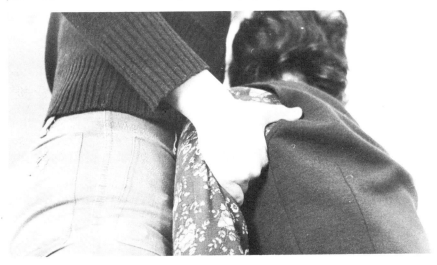

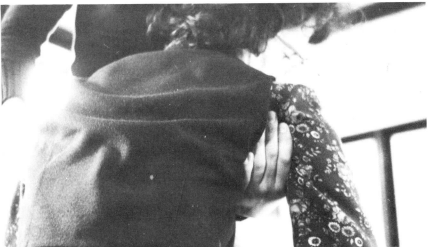

Fig. 9. *The armpit hold.* Top: *the arm which holds from the back.* Bottom: *the arm which goes across the front.* Note: *the fingers go right through the armpit and the thumbs are left outside*

8. Elbow grip

The helper stands as for the pelvic hold and moves the handicapped person near to the front edge of the chair. She takes a firm stance so that her forward foot and knee block the handicapped person's foot and knee. Her weight should be taken on this leg.

The helper leans the handicapped person forward from the hips with as straight a back as possible. She grasps the near elbow with the adjacent hand and reaches across the back of the neck and in front of the far shoulder to grasp the far elbow. *Note that no pressure should be exerted on the neck.* The handicapped person's elbows are tucked well into his waist and kept a little to the back, and the helper then grasps under the points of the elbows so that she holds the handicapped person closely against her own body.

By rocking on her forward leg she then lifts the handicapped person by the elbows (Fig. 10).

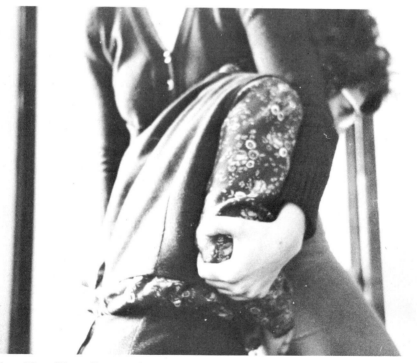

Fig. 10. *The elbow grip: the handicapped person is leaned forward.* Above: *the hands grasp each elbow.* Opposite: *a general view to show how to reach across the neck and in front of the shoulders*

18

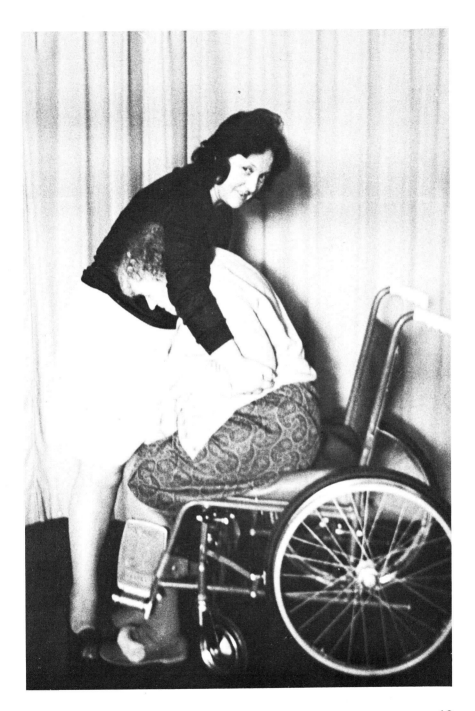

9. Holds for adjusting the handicapped person's position

When helping the handicapped person to adjust his position by moving a limb, the helper's hand must be placed underneath the part to be lifted and the whole palmar surface used to support rather than grip the part.

When adjusting the position of the body or both legs together it is advisable to use the whole of the forearm as well as the hand.

On all occasions when lifting a heavy person or taking heavy pressure, the helper's elbow must be tucked into her waist, so that some of the strain is taken through her upright body, to the strong muscles of the legs.

Basic Lifts for Helpers

These are as follows:

1. Orthodox lift.
2. Shoulder lift.
3. Modified shoulder lift.
4. Through-arm lift.
5. Elbow lift.
6. Three-man lift.

In all lifting it is essential for the helpers and, where applicable, the handicapped person to synchronise their efforts. Good timing is achieved with practice but it is necessary for one helper to assume control and give the instructions when to lift. It may be necessary to make several attempts in some moves and lifts by building up momentum, as in swinging on a garden swing.

The lift should be planned beforehand and everyone should know what is happening.

To prevent accidents the area should be cleared and the necessary furniture secured so that it does not move at the vital moment.

1. Orthodox lift

This lift may be used in most circumstances and requires two helpers. It has the advantage that the helpers can observe the handicapped person's face. It is more difficult than the shoulder lift for the helpers to achieve without strain, especially when starting from and/or finishing in a low position and when lifting heavy people. However, it is to be preferred when the handicapped person has very weak shoulder muscles or where there is a painful condition of the shoulders or chest wall.

The helpers' feet are positioned as near to the handicapped person as possible, standing astride with one foot facing the direction of movement. The helpers stand facing each other with their knees and hips bent, their backs straight and their heads held up. Their hands are inserted under the handicapped person's thighs as near to his hips as possible, and the wrist or finger grip is used (Figs. 2 and 3, pp. 12, 13). The handicapped person's arms may be round the helpers' shoulders. The helpers' hands at the back should be as low as possible.

(a) *Lifting up on a high bed.* The handicapped person should be instructed to keep his chin in. When a lift up the bed is required, where possible he should be encouraged to assist by pushing with his heels and straightening his knees.

The helpers achieve the lift by straightening their knees and hips (Fig. 11). They move the handicapped person by transferring their weight from one foot to the other in the desired direction.

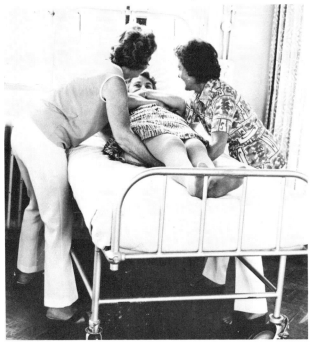

Fig. 11. *The orthodox lift: lifting up a high bed. The handicapped person must lift the head slightly*

(b) *Adaptation of the lift for use on a low bed.* When lifting a handicapped person up a low bed it is difficult to employ the orthodox lift unless a draw sheet or roller towel is used (Fig. 12). Note that a firm grip is taken on the sheet (as close as possible to the handicapped person).

(c) *Lifting from bed to chair or from chair to bed.* As soon as the handicapped person is clear of the bed, the helpers transfer some of their weight to the forward foot (Fig. 13), so that their weight is equally distributed between their feet. The helpers stay as close to the handicapped person as possible. When lowering him into a chair, the helpers' backs remain straight and their hips and knees bend.

2. Shoulder lift

This lift may be used in most situations and is of particular help when lifting heavy people.

The helpers have one relatively free hand, which, when it is not supporting the handicapped person's back, can be used to push on or steady the furniture, and even to open a door.

It is valuable when carrying someone over a distance as the helpers are facing the direction in which they are travelling, and it can be used on stairs.

The lift may need to be modified when there is a pain problem in the shoulders or chest wall, and if the handicapped person has no power in his shoulders or arms.

To prepare for the lift:

(a) The handicapped person sits as upright as possible.

(b) The helpers stand shoulder to shoulder with, and slightly behind, the handicapped person, as close to the bed or chair as possible, feet astride with the forward foot facing the direction of movement.

(c) The helpers bend at the hips and knees, keeping their backs straight and heads up.

(d) The helpers press their near shoulders into the handicapped person's chest wall under the armpit so that his arms may rest on their backs.

(e) The helpers' hands are placed under the thighs as near the buttocks as possible. The wrist or finger grip is used, but for obese

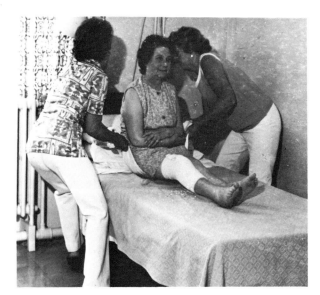

Fig. 12. *The orthodox lift: adaptation for a low bed using a draw sheet or roller towel*

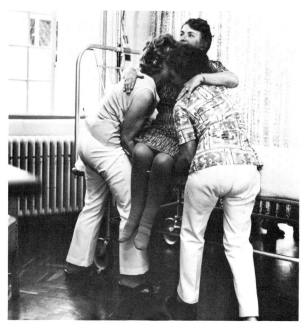

Fig. 13. *The orthodox lift: lifting from bed to chair or vice versa*

persons the hand might be placed palm up under the adjacent thigh. The lift is achieved by the helpers straightening their hips and knees (Fig. 14).

3. Modified shoulder lift
If the arms tend to move so that the armpit is no longer a niche into which the lifter's shoulder can be placed, the disabled person's arms can be held as in Fig. 15. The instructions above are followed until the helpers' shoulders are inserted under the armpit and then the disabled person's forearms are hooked so that each is held between the helpers' arm and chest. The helpers' hands are then

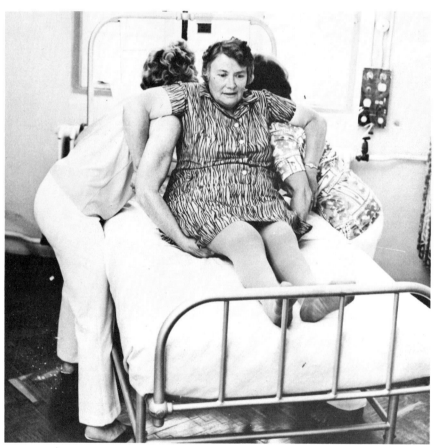

Fig. 14.   *The shoulder lift: lifting up a high bed. The handicapped person's arms may rest on the helpers' backs*

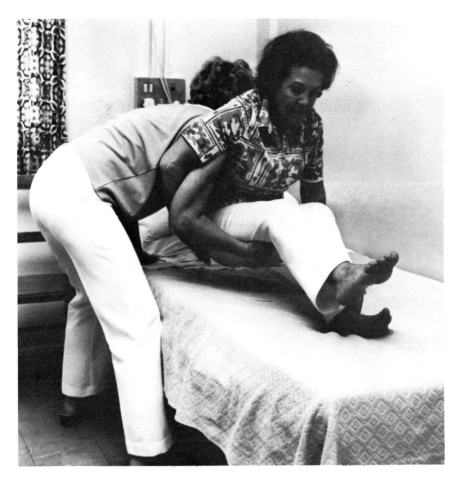

Fig. 15.   *The modified shoulder lift: the handicapped person's arm is held between the helper's chest wall and upper arm*

placed under the thighs as high as possible. The modification also allows a very obese person to be lifted, as the helpers need not grip each other's hands under the thighs but can each put their hands palm up under the thighs.

Either the shoulder lift or the modified shoulder lift can be used as follows when:

(a) *Lifting on a high bed*. The helpers' hands are on the bed ready to assist the lift. The handicapped person should be instructed to keep his chin in. When a lift up the bed is required he should be encouraged to assist by pushing with his feet and straightening his knees.

The helpers prepare to lift by pressing their shoulders into the chest wall. To lift the handicapped person clear of the bed, they straighten their legs and push on the free arm simultaneously. The move up the bed is brought about by transferring the weight from one foot to the other in the desired direction (Fig. 14).

(b) *Lifting on a low single bed*. The rear knee of each helper is placed on the bed level with the handicapped person's hips (Fig. 16). The helpers sit on their heels with the foot of the kneeling leg over the side of the bed. To lift, the helpers thrust with their legs, straightening their knees. This lifts the handicapped person and carries him up the bed.

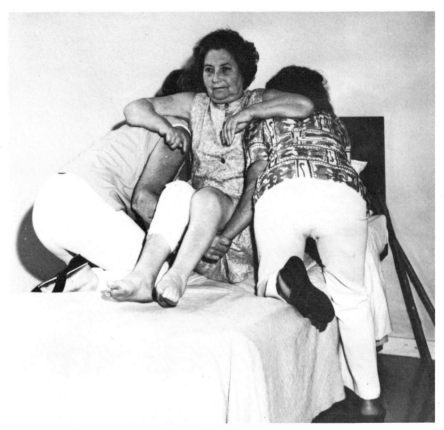

Fig. 16.   *The shoulder lift: lifting on a low single bed*

(c) *Lifting on a low double bed.* The handicapped person is first moved towards the side of the bed to enable one helper to take up the same position as for lifting in a low single bed. The second helper must get on the bed and kneel at the side of the handicapped person.

(d) *Lifting from bed to chair or from chair to bed* (Figs. 17(a) and (b)). The handicapped person should, if possible, be near to the front of the chair or bed to enable the helpers to get their hands under his thighs in a wrist grip. The arms of a wheelchair may be removed. In order to lift, the helpers should push with their free hands on the arms or back of the seat of the chair or on the bed to assist the

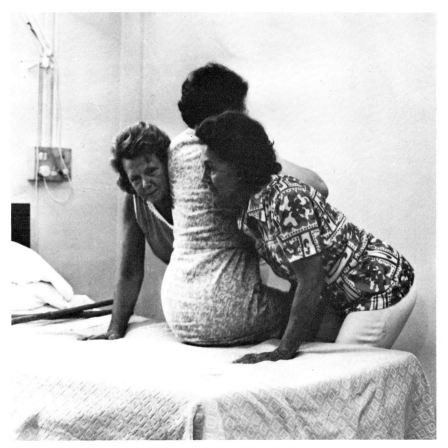

Fig. 17(a). *The shoulder lift: lifting from bed in sitting position. The start or finish*

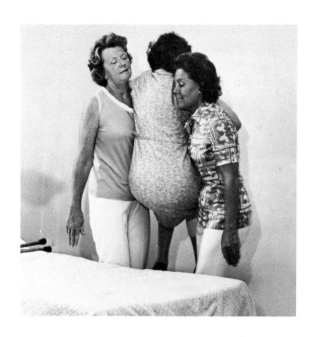

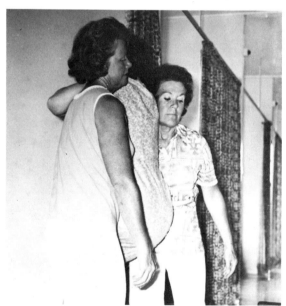

Fig. 17(b).　*The shoulder lift: lifting from bed in
sitting position.* Top: *the carrying position.*
Bottom: *the helpers each have a free hand*

28

upwards thrust of their legs. *When carrying, the helpers' hands may need to support the handicapped person's back, or may be free to carry something or to open a door.*

(e) *Lifting from the floor.* The position of the helpers' legs is important. They may choose either to kneel on the knee nearer to the handicapped person or to have both knees bent in the curtsey sitting or crouch position. In either case the outer foot is in front of the nearer knee or foot. This is a difficult lift and helpers may find the through-arm lift easier—*see* p. 30.

(f) *Lowering to the floor.* The shoulder lift (Figs. 18(a) and (b)) may be used here but it is probable that the through-arm lift will prove easier.

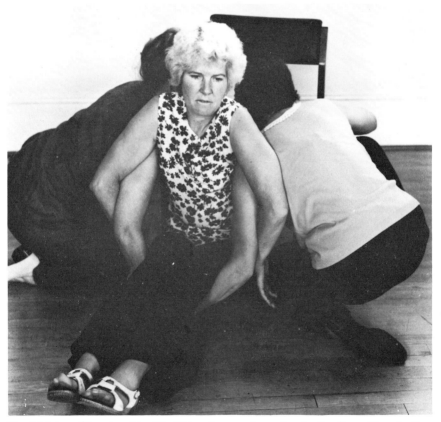

Fig. 18(a).   *The shoulder lift: lifting from or lowering to the floor. The starting position*

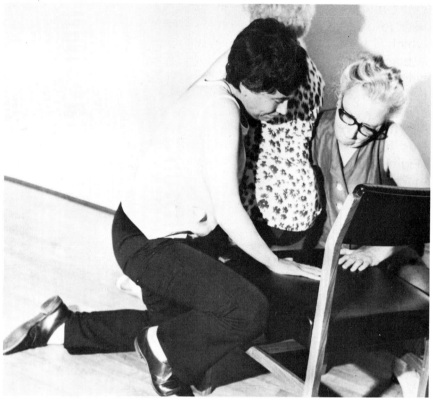

Fig. 18(b). *The shoulder lift: lifting from or lowering to the floor. The lift almost completed*

4. Through-arm lift

This lift is most effective when the helper at the head can get directly behind the handicapped person and if possible stand or kneel above him. The lift is very useful when lifting from or to a low position as it is easy for the helper to maintain an upright back.

In the carrying position there is very close contact between the handicapped person and the helper at the head end. Thus much of the weight is transmitted directly to the floor.

The handicapped person should have some power in one arm and hand (Fig. 4) so that he can grasp his weaker wrist with the stronger hand. The helper puts her hands through between his chest and arms from behind, and grasps the handicapped person's arms as near his wrists as possible.

(a) *Lifting up on the bed.* The handicapped person should be near to one side of the bed. The helper kneels "up" on the knee which is placed on the bed. To allow room for the move the knee is placed a short distance behind the handicapped person as the helper sits behind him. The grip is as in Fig. 4, p. 13. The move is achieved by the helper thrusting back with the standing leg. At the end of the lift the helper is sitting back on the heel of the kneeling leg. If possible the handicapped person can help by bending his legs and thrusting at the same time by pushing on his heels (Fig. 19). If a second helper is needed, the lift will be as illustrated in Fig. 20.

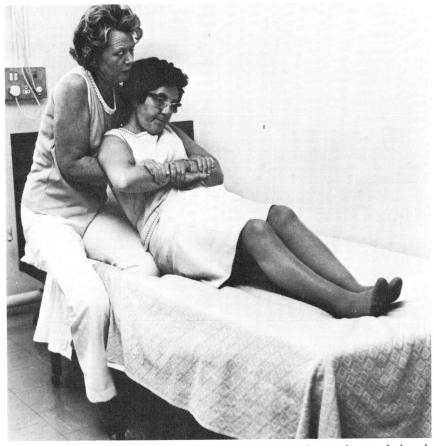

Fig. 19.   *The through-arm lift: lifting up the bed when only one helper is available*

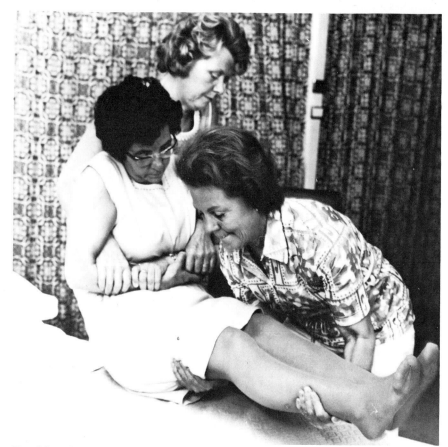

Fig. 20.   *The through-arm lift: lifting up the bed with a second helper lifting the legs*

(b) *Lifting from or to seats of similar heights, e.g. bed, chair, W.C.*
The helper at the head may not be able to stand directly behind the chair. To avoid the arm of the chair either the handicapped person must be positioned well forward at the edge of the chair or he will have to be lifted forward.

If the arm of the wheelchair can be removed the handicapped person can be lifted sideways; if not he can be lifted forward by slight adjustment of the helper's starting position. The helper may have to stand to the side.

When planning the lift, the helper lifting the legs must select the side on which to stand so that she does not find herself between the bed and the person she is lifting. The helper lifting the legs must support the handicapped person's thighs. Her knees and hips must be fully bent and her back straight. The helpers hold the handicapped person closely into their bodies.

If the bed is slightly higher than the general level of the lift, the handicapped person may be raised to the required height by a swinging movement. This will require practice and two people who are accustomed to working together.

(c) *Lifting from the floor*

(i) *On to a seat*. The helper at the head should be directly behind the handicapped person and very close to his back. The second

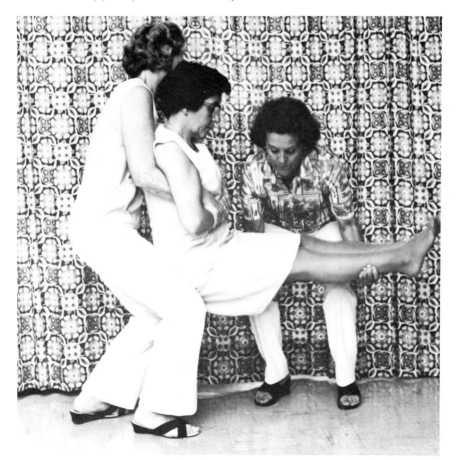

Fig. 21. *The through-arm lift: lifting from the floor in the sitting position*

helper lifts the legs, supporting them at the knees and ankles. Both helpers must bend their knees and hips to take hold and then straighten their legs in order to lift (Fig. 21).

(ii) *Into standing position*. It may be necessary to fix the feet either against a wall or with the assistance of a second helper. Where possible the handicapped person's knees should be fully bent with his feet flat on the floor. This lift may also be used if the legs are fixed straight by calipers. In this case the feet *must* be fixed. In all situations the helper's back remains upright and the work is done by the strong leg muscles (Fig. 22).

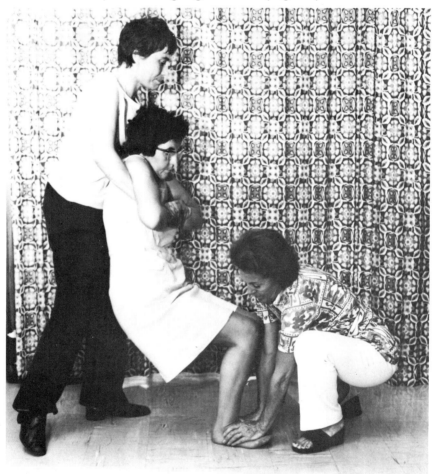

Fig. 22.   *The through-arm lift: lifting from the floor into standing*

(d) *Lifting the sitting handicapped person into a good position well back into the wheelchair.* First of all, sit the handicapped person in an upright position. The helper stands behind the chair and takes a through-arm grasp. If necessary a second person can lift the legs in the usual way.

5. Elbow lift

This is an original lift invented to allow a disabled person to be lifted by one person and rotated through 180° before being sat down again. It is especially useful when transferring a helpless person from wheelchair to W.C. seat in a confined space, *e.g.* when chair and W.C. face one another. It can also be used through 90° and is feasible even from a fixed-arm wheelchair or chair to another seat.

The helper stands on the side opposite to the direction of the turn. The handicapped person is moved near the front edge of the seat. The foot-rests on the wheelchair must be lifted. The helper's forward foot is placed to block the handicapped person's feet inside the wheelchair area. The handicapped person's knees are blocked by the knee of this leg. The helper's other leg is outside the side of the wheelchair (*see* Fig. 10, p. 19). The handicapped person is leaned forward and the helper puts the upper part of her adjacent arm around the back of his neck and leans forward to grasp under the points of both elbows. The furthermost arm, as shown in Fig. 10, p. 18, is in front of the shoulder and the adjacent shoulder is held firm against the helper's body. The helper pulls in the line of the handicapped person's back, using the fixed forward knee and foot as a pivot. *No attempt* is made to lift in one go. The lift is a series of rocking movements of the handicapped person's body, his buttocks lifting higher each time, and eventually high enough for a turn/pivot to be executed by the helper pulling a little harder on the furthermost arm. If the handicapped person's feet tend to cross and lock, so obstructing the turn, they should be crossed at the ankle before the lift begins. The leg further from the helper should be crossed in front of the nearer leg.

6. Three-man total lift

It may be necessary to lift a very handicapped person from or to a trolley or wheelchair. This usually needs three people (Fig. 23).

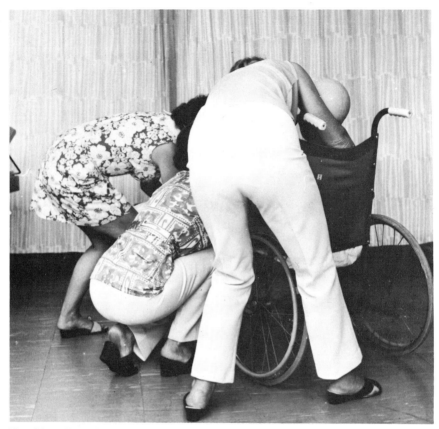

Fig. 23. *The three-man lift from a chair.* Above: *preparation.* Opposite, top: *the lift completed and the helpers ready to move.* Opposite, bottom: *lowering on to a trolley*

(a) *Lifting a person of average weight.* The three helpers arrange themselves alongside the trolley or chair facing the handicapped person. The most experienced takes the head and shoulders. The handicapped person's arms are placed across his body and one leg is crossed over the other. The helper at the head places her nearest arm as far as possible round the handicapped person's shoulders, resting his head in the crook of her arm. The other arm is placed as far under the body as possible at waist level. The helper in the middle places one arm at waist level next to the first helper and the other arm under the thighs. The helper at the foot end places her arms under the legs. To get the arms as far through as required it is

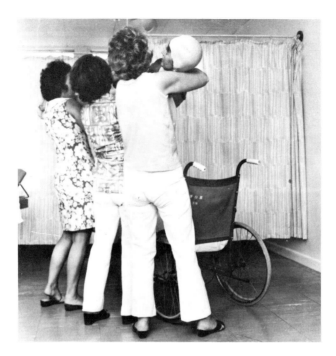

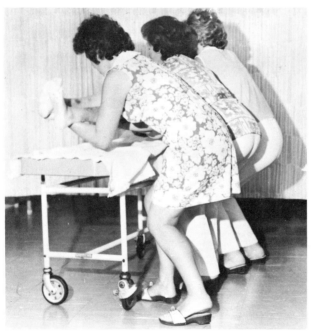

necessary for the helpers to be standing with one foot in advance of the other, the forward knee bent and the rear leg straight. The lifter at the head gives the order to lift, and the handicapped person is lifted clear of the trolley. The helpers use their legs to lift and at the same time roll the handicapped person towards themselves (Fig. 23, p. 37 *top*), and on to their chests so that the weight is taken through the body and directly over the feet.

This lift is suitable for transferring a handicapped person from a trolley or chair to a high-level bed or on to a hoist for lowering into a pool. It must be planned carefully beforehand. The lifters must know the direction of movement to be taken following the lift.

(b) *Transferring a heavy person directly from a lying position on to a trolley or chair.* The lifters arrange themselves as in method (a) but the helper at the head end uses the through-arm lift grasp. The lifter in the middle who has a considerable part of the weight must ensure that she holds the handicapped person closely to her body. It is essential that the chair is secure and will not move, and where possible the chair arm should be removed. The chair must be angled towards the trolley but far enough away to give the lifters room to move. The lifters at the hips and legs must keep their backs straight as they lower the handicapped person into the chair.

Chapter 4

GENERAL MOBILITY

P. J. Waddington, M.C.S.P., Dip.T.P.
M. Hollis, M.B.E., M.C.S.P., Dip.T.P.

It is important for the handicapped person's psychological and physical needs for him to be as mobile and independent as possible. A fully rehabilitated person is one who needs little or no help from others to perform his daily tasks.

This section is designed to give the helper some insight into some well-tried ways in which the handicapped person may practise independence, and to indicate the ways in which help may be given when necessary.

Two Basic Transfer Movements

In all well co-ordinated activities, the body moves in one of two ways:

1. *Straight movement* either forward, when the head must move first, or backward, when the buttocks should move first (Fig. 24).

2. *Sideways movement with rotation*, when the same rule applies but the head and buttocks move simultaneously in opposite directions (Fig. 25).

Before using either movement, the handicapped person lifts his hips clear. There is an arc of movement on the swing which helps to clear obstructions. If the handicapped person cannot lift himself clear he can practise by placing each hand on a wooden block or thick book (Fig. 26). This gives more thrust from the slightly bent elbow. As well as giving the feeling of the movement, this exercises the elbow and shoulder muscles.

Use of a Sliding Board

If the handicapped person cannot lift his weight on his arms or if the distance between the transfer points is too great, he may find a sliding board useful (Fig. 27).

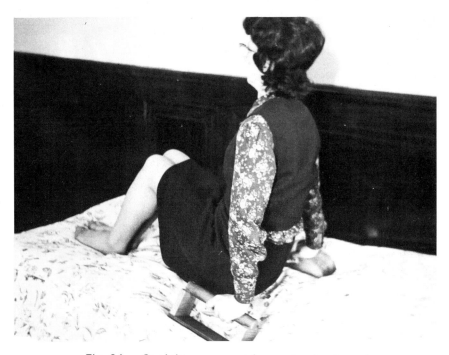

Fig. 24. *Straight movement forward or backward*

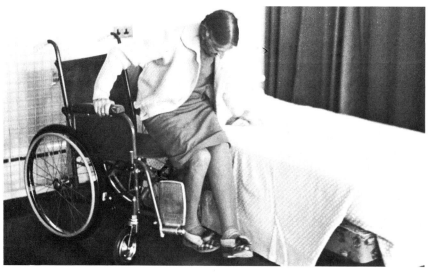

Fig. 25. *Sideways movement with rotation: the hips and head move in opposite directions*

40

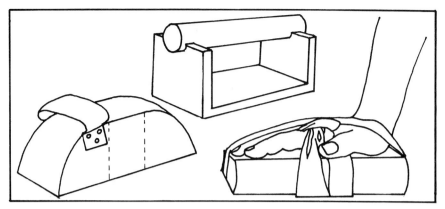

Fig. 26. *The blocks which can be used to lengthen the arms.* Left: *a wooden block 8 in. (20 cm) long by 3½ in. (9 cm) wide and 2¾ in. (7·5 cm) deep, rounded at the ends but with a central flat part on top about 2 in. (5 cm) long. Velcro is attached to the block towards the front so that the block can be fixed across the fingers.* Centre: *a handle 1½ in. (4 cm) in diameter mounted on blocks of wood about 3¼ in. (8·5 cm) high by 3¾ in. (9·5 cm) wide with a base plate 8 in. (20 cm) long by 3¾ in. (9·5 cm) wide.* Right: *a thick book*

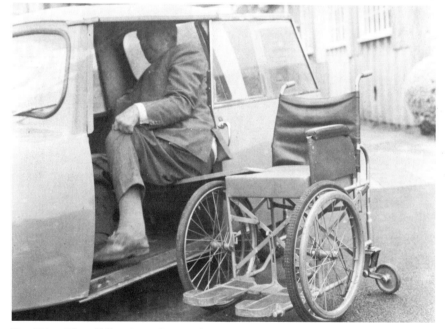

Fig. 27. *The sliding board: used for transferring over a greater distance than the handicapped person can reach*

The board should be highly polished and have bevelled edges. It should not be heavy, and should be made either out of strong wood such as mahogany or out of chipboard, covered with a thin layer of foam, covered again with Fablon and polished. It should measure about $\frac{1}{2}$ in. (1·5 cm) thick and 10–12 in. (25–30 cm) wide. The length will vary according to the purpose; *e.g.* a board used for transfers from chair to car needs to be longer than one used from bed to chair.

The handicapped person places one end of the board under his seat and ensures that the other end is resting securely in position. The helper, if needed, should stand at the back.

Functional Activities

These are as follows:

1. Moving to the side of the bed.
2. Turning in bed.
3. Sitting and moving up the bed.
4. Sitting on the side of the bed.
5. Sitting to sitting.
6. Standing from sitting.
7. Sitting from standing.
8. Sitting to the floor.
9. Floor to chair.
10. Assisted walking.
11. Basic movement when using axillary (underarm) crutches.
12. Carrying a child.
13. Wheelchair and stairs.
14. Emergency situations.

1. Moving to the side of the bed
It may be necessary for the handicapped person, before attempting to sit, to move towards the side of the bed.

(a) *Without help*

(i) In the lying position with his knees bent so that his feet are flat on the bed, the handicapped person raises his hips by pressing on his heels and shoulders, and moves the buttocks sideways. The legs and head and shoulder can then follow.

(ii) If he is in the sitting position the handicapped person can raise his hips by pressing on his hands and feet with his knee or knees bent. By putting one hand far enough away from the side of his body he can move his hips sideways or turn slightly as he does so.

(b) *With help.* The handicapped person is moved in three stages (Fig. 28):

Stage 1. The legs are moved. The helper places one knee on the bed, places her hands under the ankles, and lifts the legs towards herself.

Stage 2. The shoulders are moved. The helper faces the handicapped person, places the knee of her near leg on the bed, leaving the foot over the edge. The hands are placed under the handicapped person's shoulders; the near hand may be used to support the head. The head and shoulders are raised as the helper takes her weight backward and sits on her heel.

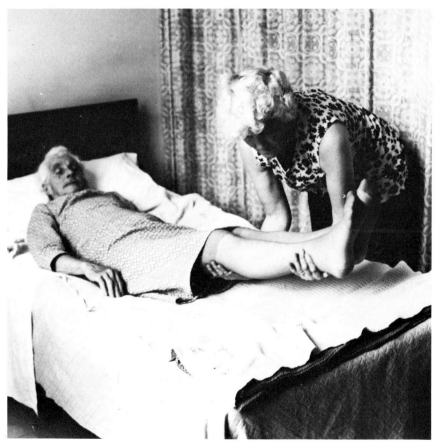

Fig. 28. *Moving to the side of the bed.* Above: *legs.* Overleaf, top: *head and shoulders.* Overleaf, bottom: *hips*

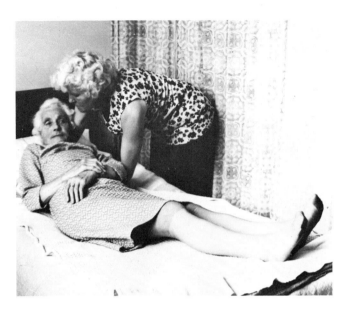

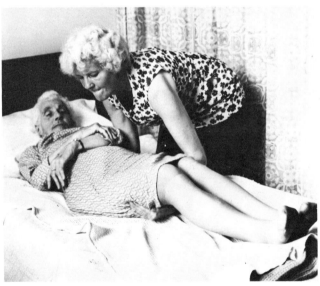

Stage 3. The hips are moved. The helper stands opposite the handicapped person's hips facing the bed, and kneels on the bed with one knee. She places one hand and arm under the waist and the other under the thighs. The hips are raised and moved as the helper carries her weight backward to sit on her heel.

2. Turning in bed

The handicapped person will find moving in bed easier if he has a firm mattress. If the mattress is soft it can be put on a piece of hardboard.

(a) *Without help.* Repeated movements, each bigger than the last, may be necessary to build up enough momentum or swing to achieve the turn.

(i) *Paralysed on one side*

1. *To the affected side.* With his normal hand, the handicapped person places his paralysed arm by his side. The normal leg is placed across the affected leg. With his normal arm across his body he grasps the mattress and, lifting his head and shoulders, he turns by pulling himself towards the affected side (Fig. 29).

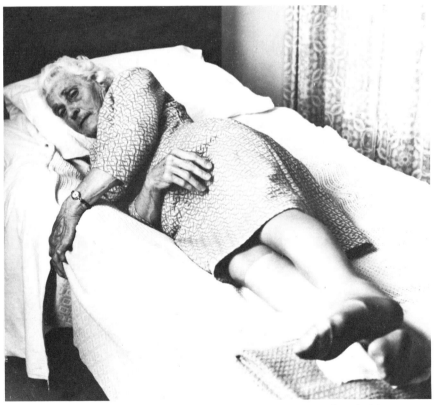

Fig. 29. *Turning in bed without help to the paralysed side*

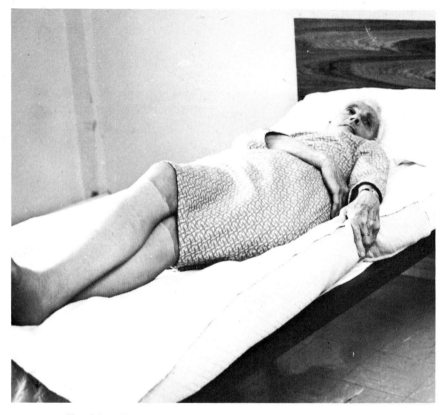

Fig. 30.   *Turning in bed without help to the normal side*

2. *To the normal side.* The handicapped person crosses his affected leg over the normal leg by lifting it with his normal hand, by pulling on his trouser leg or by slipping his normal foot under the affected leg at the ankle. He lifts his affected arm across his body (Fig. 30). He grasps the mattress with his normal hand at that side and, raising his head and shoulder, he pulls himself over.

(ii) *Paralysed below the waist.* The method used is basically the same as above. The handicapped person has to lift one leg over the other; *e.g.* turning to the left the right leg is uppermost and vice versa. He turns by pulling with the near hand and pushing with the hand away from the turn.

(b) *With help.* It may be necessary to lift the handicapped person to the side of the bed by lifting the legs, the head and shoulders, and finally the buttocks (Fig. 28, pp. 43, 44). The arm and leg of the

46

same side are crossed over towards the direction of the roll. The helper, who is as near to the handicapped person as possible, gets down, if the bed is low, by bending one knee and placing it on the bed, thus keeping the back straight (Fig. 31). When rolling the handicapped person away from herself the helper's knees are bent (*i.e.* that on the bed and that on which she stands). To complete the turn she pushes with her standing leg, and straightens the knee. With palm upwards the helper's hands and forearms are placed as far as possible under the handicapped person's shoulder and hip. When rolling the handicapped person towards herself the

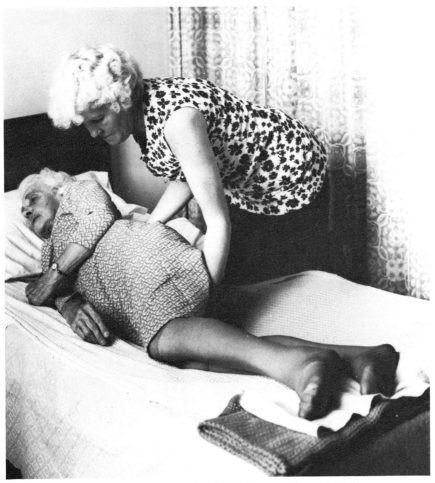

Fig. 31. *Turning in bed with help away from the helper*

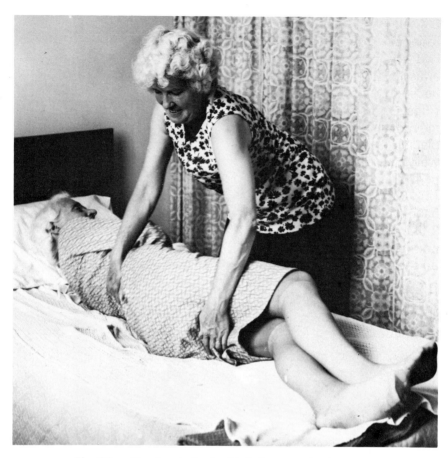

Fig. 32. *Turning in bed with help towards the helper*

helper starts with her weight well forward over the bent knee on the bed with the rear standing leg straight (Fig. 32). By bending both knees and moving backward the helper uses her body weight to turn the handicapped person. The helper's hands are placed comfortably on the far side of the handicapped person's shoulder and hip.

3. Sitting and moving up the bed
(a) *Without help*

(i) *Straight movement.* This method is suitable for people with good use of both arms. If the handicapped person cannot push himself into the sitting position in the normal way, he may find a rope, either knotted or with a handle, attached to the foot of the bed useful for pulling himself up into sitting. He should keep his arms low near the thighs and raise his head first. When upright he should support himself by propping with arms behind him (Figs. 33(a) and (b)). Having attained the sitting position he can move himself straight backwards. If he cannot clear the bed when placing his hands palm downwards he can make a fist and put his weight through his knuckles, or use the hand blocks (Fig. 24, p. 40).

(ii) *Sideways movement with rotation.* (Fig. 25, p. 40). The handicapped person turns on to his normal side as described in **2** above. He pushes himself up on to his elbows. Having bent his normal knee, he uses his elbow and leg to lift his hips and move them up the bed.

(b) *With help*

(i) *Sitting.* The helper kneels on the bed with her near knee facing the handicapped person. She keeps her weight forward. The

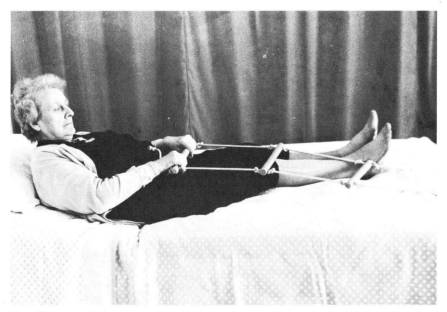

Fig. 33(a). *Sitting up using a "ladder" rope.* Note: *the head must be lifted first*

49

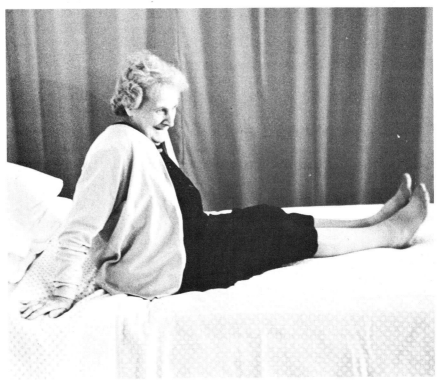

Fig. 33(b).   *Sitting: propping with arms behind*

helper has one hand behind the handicapped person's shoulder and the other at the nape of his neck. The handicapped person can assist by pushing with the hand furthest away from the helper.

(ii) *Moving up the bed.* The modification of the shoulder lift makes it perfectly possible to use this lift on a person with a severely disabled side (arm and leg) and allows him to thrust with his sound bent knee and a hand block (Fig. 15, p. 25) held slightly behind him if moving up the bed. The helper takes up the position for the modified shoulder lift and gives the command *"Push!"* As the shoulder lift is applied, the disabled person thrusts and helps. It may be better to progress a little at a time up or down the bed, in which case the sound hand and leg position should be re-adjusted after each movement.

The through-arm lift with the helper on the bed can also be used (Figs. 19 and 20, pp. 31, 32).

4. Sitting on the side of the bed

(a) *Without help*

(i) The sitting person who has good power in his arms will have little difficulty in lifting his legs over the side of the bed. If his balance is poor he may need to support himself on one hand throughout.

(ii) *Weakness down one side*

1. *Towards the affected side.* The handicapped person lifts his affected leg over the side of the bed and follows it with his normal leg. He leans forward and, pushing with his hand, turns towards the side of the bed. He may need to support himself with his normal hand and arm.

2. *Towards the non-affected side.* The affected arm is put across the body. The normal foot is pushed under the ankle of the weaker leg. The handicapped person, by pushing on the normal arm and lifting the normal leg together, can swing into the sitting position on the side of the bed. Alternatively the normal leg is placed over the side of the bed and the weaker leg lifted over by hand.

(b) *With help*

(i) The handicapped person is first sat up and held upright by one hand behind the shoulder. The legs are lifted to and over the side of the bed and the handicapped person is pivoted by pressure on the shoulder. If he has any arm or leg ability he should assist with appropriate thrusting actions.

(ii) The modified shoulder lift can be used if the helper stands at the disabled side and the handicapped person pushes on a hand block and his sound heel. The weaker leg is moved first either to or over the side of the bed, and then a combined thrust can pivot the disabled person so that he turns towards the side of the bed. Two lifts are usually necessary to complete the turn.

(iii) With the handicapped person lying near to the edge of the bed, it is possible, depending upon relative size, for a helper to swing him into a sitting position over the side of the bed in one movement (Fig. 34). The helper places one hand under the nape of the neck, the other under the knees, and pivots him round on his hips.

5. Sitting to sitting

(a) *Bed to chair or chair to bed.* For handicapped people with adequate use of both arms either the straight transfer forward or the sideways transfer with rotation may be used (*see* p. 40).

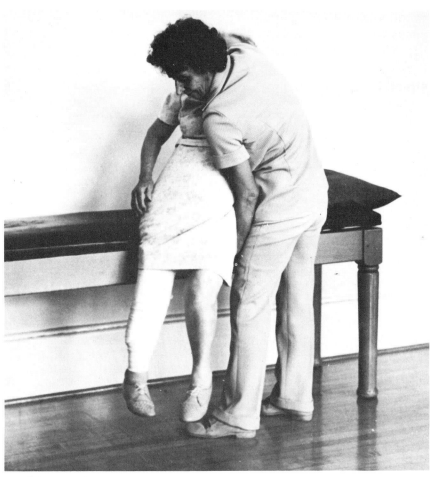

Fig. 34. *A tall helper pivoting a handicapped person from lying to sitting on the edge of the bed ready for standing*

(i) *Straight transfer forward to and from a wheelchair.* The chair is drawn up facing the bed and as close as possible. The foot-rests may have to be the type that swing backward. The brake of the wheelchair must be firmly on.

Difficulty is sometimes experienced when transferring straight forward from chair to bed because the heels may become caught up in the sheet. A zip-backed chair is then indicated to *allow straight transfer backward.* This backward transfer is the method of choice for the person with both legs amputated, who may be able to turn round within the confines of the chair seat. He can then come out backward from a chair drawn up to face the bed (Fig. 24, p. 40). (ii) *Sideways transfer with rotation*. This is often more useful for those paralysed from the waist down. In many cases transfers are easier if the chair is slightly angled towards the bed. This is particularly so if a helper is needed and/or the chair has a fixed arm (Fig. 25, p. 40).

Otherwise a chair with removable arms is positioned either parallel with or at a slight angle to the bed (a sliding board may be used). After the chair arm has been removed, the handicapped person lifts his legs on to the bed—he may need help. He then places one hand on the bed, the other on the chair, and thrusts, lifting his hips clear. Simultaneously he rotates his hips, the arc of movement clearing the wheel. If required, the helper stands behind the handicapped person between the bed and the chair and helps by lifting the hips from the waist.

Figure 35 shows a sideways transfer from wheelchair to bed.

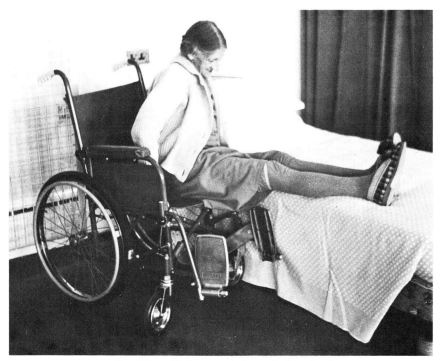

Fig. 35. *Sitting to sitting: chair to bed*

Note the position of the chair (brakes on). The handicapped person first lifts the legs on to the bed and uses a sideways movement to transfer the hips. If necessary a helper can stand behind the handicapped person between the bed and the chair in a position to help lift the legs over.

When a handicapped person who has weakness down one side is sitting on the side of the bed, the chair is placed at the person's useful side and at a slight angle towards the bed. If a wheelchair is used, the foot-rests are lifted up and the brakes are put on.

1. *From sitting to sitting.* From the sitting position the handicapped person reaches across to the far arm of the chair, takes the weight on the useful leg and swings into the chair in one movement.

2. *Sitting through standing to sitting.* The handicapped person stands and then reaches for the far arm of the chair, rotates the hips and sits down. If a helper is required she can stand in front so that she is in a position to block the weaker knee and assist in standing by holding the waistband or belt.

3. *Armpit hold and swing.* The helper stands obliquely with forward foot and knee to block the paralysed leg. The handicapped person may sit nearer the front edge of the chair and leans forwards from the hips. He uses his able hand to push on the chair arm or seat or the bed or his own thigh. The helper takes the armpit hold (Fig. 9, p. 17) and gives the command: *"Push!"* Together the disabled person pushing on the sound leg and hand, and the helper lifting obliquely forward and upward in the line of the back, make several attempts at rising. At a sufficiently high point in the swing the helper exerts a rotating pressure so that the disabled person is turned to allow his buttocks to be over the new seat as he descends from the last upswing.

(b) *Chair to car.* Note that the use of "right" and "left" refers to the front passenger seat of a right-hand-drive car.

The same basic principles apply here as for all transfer activities. The use of a sliding board may make this manoeuvre easier and is essential for some people (Fig. 27, p. 41).

The car door should be opened wide and the windows wound down to enable the handicapped person to grip the frame. The brakes of the wheelchair must be on and the chair conveniently near to the car. Care must be taken by the handicapped person not to hit his head.

Although it is usual for a handicapped person to sit in the front seat of a car, it is possible to get him into the rear seat of a four-door car.

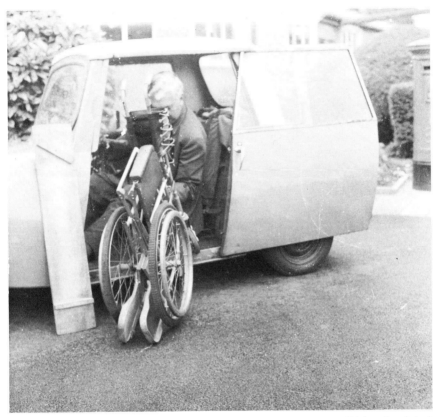

Fig. 36. *After transferring to the car, a strong person can pull his wheelchair into the car*

With the right vehicle many well-balanced and strong people can pull the folded wheelchair into the car (Fig. 36).

(i) *Straight backward.* As before, this method is of use to the person with both legs amputated and to the person paralysed below the waist (paraplegic) with weak arms. The wheelchair will have a zipped back, and a sliding board may prove useful.

(ii) *Sideways with rotation.* This may be done in two ways:

1. *Sitting to sitting.* The young strong paraplegic will be able to do this without difficulty; other people will need a sliding board. It is usual for the handicapped person to get his hips into the car first and follow them with his legs, and to lift the legs out of the car first, followed by his hips. However, the reverse method may prove to be easier.

55

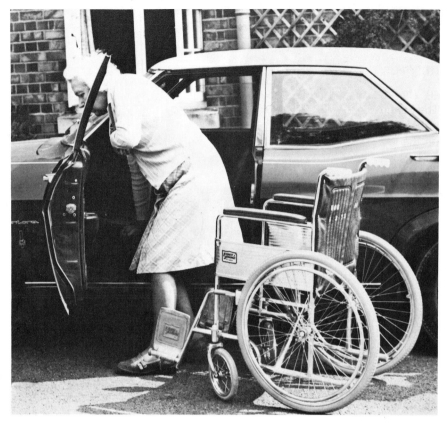

Fig. 37. *Transferring by sideways movement with rotation from wheelchair to car seat, through standing*

2. *Sitting through standing to sitting.* This method is likely to be used by the person with weakness down one side. The chair should be positioned so that the handicapped person can make full use of the normal side (Fig. 37).

(a) *Person with weakness down the left side.*

(i) *Into the car (front passenger seat).* The chair is drawn up at an angle to the car. The handicapped person twists in his chair so that he can grip the car door (window down). He stands. He twists a little further and sits down backward on to the car seat. He can then get his legs into the car.

(ii) *Out of the car (front passenger seat).* The chair is drawn up parallel to the car door (window down). The handicapped person lifts his left leg out of the car, following it with his right. He may either grip the car door and stand, or rotate in the seat so that he can reach for and grip the right arm of the chair. He turns in the standing position, grasps the right arm of the chair and sits down. From the twisted sitting position he takes weight on his leg and arm, rotates further and sits in a semi-flexed position.

(b) *Person with weakness down the right side.*

(i) *Into the car (front passenger seat).* The chair is up level with the car door. The handicapped person grips either the car door or chair arm to aid standing, grips the back of the car seat or stanchion (back window wound down), pivots on the left leg and sits down backward. He takes the weight on the left leg and arm, stands, rotates and sits down backward. Then he lifts his legs into the car.

(ii) *Out of the car (front passenger seat).* The chair is drawn up parallel with the car door. The handicapped person lifts both legs out of the car. Either he winds the back window down, grips the stanchion and stands, turns and sits down, or he rotates in the seat and reaches for the left arm of the chair, takes his weight on the left leg and arm, pivots on the leg and sits down.

(c) *Chair to W.C.* The basic transfer methods with or without help apply here. The method selected will depend upon the handicapped person's abilities; the space available; the adaptation made to the W.C. seat and the availability of suitable hand-rails.

Suitable methods may be as follows:

(i) *Transfer from chair to W.C. through standing.* Even in a confined space this should present no difficulty if the basic principles are applied and hand-rails provided (*see* **6** below).

(ii) *Direct transfers.* If the room is wide enough the chair can be drawn up alongside or near the W.C. and the sideways transfer made (*see* p. 39). The level of the W.C. seat may have to be adjusted to the level of the chair seat and a suitable hand-rail provided. As many W.C.s are narrow the straight transfer (*see* p. 39) will have to be used. Again the level of the W.C. seat may have to be adjusted. The backward transfer can be made with a zip-backed chair, leaving the legs on the seat of the chair for easy return. On occasions, probably in difficult circumstances, the handicapped person can transfer on to the W.C. so that he is sitting astride the pot facing the wall.

(iii) *Elbow lift* (Fig. 38). This is used when total help is needed (*see* p. 35).

(d) *Chair to bath.* There must be a non-slip mat in the bath. There should be suitable hand-rails at the side of the bath on the wall

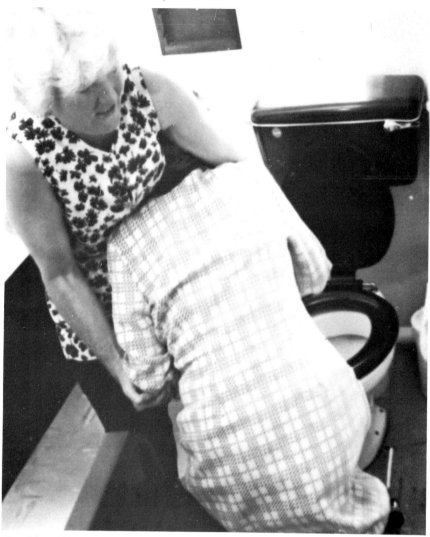

Fig. 38. *The elbow lift used for transferring a heavily handicapped person from a wheelchair to a facing W.C. in a confined space*

or attached to the taps. It may be necessary to have an overhead rope or hoist. A bath seat may be required. These are of two types:

(i) With a continuous bench seat over the bath and adjacent side and level with bath edge, and a second lower-level seat in the bath. The handicapped person transfers to the bench and moves along lifting his legs over the bath side at a suitable time. He can then transfer down on to the second level seat and so into the bath.

(ii) With a low seat inside the bath. The handicapped person sits on the side of the bath, lifts his legs over, and then lowers himself into the seat. The basic transfer methods are then used.

Getting out of the bath usually presents more problems than getting in. The water should always be let out first, then one of the above aids used. In a few cases a purpose-built shower is the only answer.

6. Standing from sitting

(a) *Unaided*. The handicapped person moves towards the front edge of the chair. His feet are pulled back as far as possible without raising the heels, and placed slightly apart. An alternative method is to place the weaker leg forward. He then leans forward keeping the head up and *either* places one hand on the arm of his chair or on the seat of an upright chair or uses his knee, and the other hand on his walking aid, *or* places both hands on the arm or seat of his chair and pushes himself upward. Alternatively, if the handicapped person can use only one hand, he should push on the chair. The walking aid is placed nearby and he changes his grasp to the aid when he has gained his balance. The height of the chair is important, as it is easier to stand from a chair with a higher seat.

(b) *With helper standing at the side*. The helper stands at the weaker side with a wide stance. She is positioned to "block" the handicapped person's weaker knee and foot. Her hips and knees are slightly bent and her back is straight (Fig. 1, p. 10).

The position of the hands may be *either* holding the nearside (weaker) arm so that she does not pull on it (Fig. 5, p. 14) *or* using the armpit hold (Fig. 39). Using either grasp she leans the handicapped person forward and assists him to stand. The helper can press forward on the bony area above the buttocks to assist the final straightening of the handicapped person.

(c) *With helper standing at the front*. The handicapped person can push on the seat or pull on a hand-rail. The helper may need to block the feet and knees with her forward leg and assist by using one of the pelvic holds.

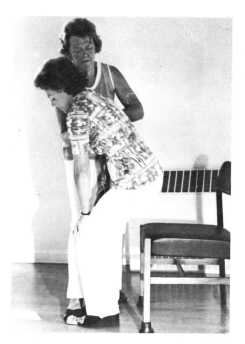

Fig. 39. *Standing with one helper blocking the feet and knee(s) and assisting using the armpit hold*

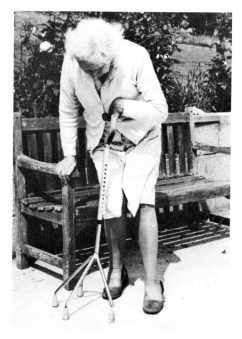

Fig. 40. *Unaided sitting by a handicapped person who is weak down one side*

(d) *With two helpers*

(i) The helpers face the handicapped person. While keeping their backs straight the helpers each position one leg to "block" the handicapped person's foot and knees on their side. The "nearer" hand is placed under the handicapped person's armpit to grasp the arm. The free hand may be used initially to push on the chair to give extra leverage; later it may be used to assist the handicapped person to extend his hips by applying pressure to the bony area above the buttocks.

(ii) With two helpers standing at the side and using the palm-to-palm grip with the forearm under the armpits, the handicapped person who has adequate arm power can press with his hands on his helpers' hands and so stand up (Fig. 6, p. 15).

7. Sitting from standing

Before sitting down it is essential for the handicapped person or helper to ensure that the chair or bed is firmly fixed. The handicapped person should always feel for the chair with the back of his legs, or look to ensure that he is at the correct distance from the seat, and then reach for the arm or seat of the chair with his hand. The handicapped person must take time about sitting. An error of judgement cannot usually be corrected once he has committed himself to "going down".

(a) *The handicapped person with adequate balance and use in both arms* usually has no difficulty in sitting. If he uses walking aids they can both be transferred to one hand while he is turning and grasping the chair with the other hand, or alternatively, laying the walking aids aside, he can grasp both arms of the chair.

If balance is poor he can be assisted either from the side, or from the front using the double forearm grasp.

(b) *Unaided sitting by the handicapped person who is weak down one side.* He stands with his back to the chair, and slightly turned towards the normal side. He looks and puts his good hand on the chair arm or bends to place his hand on the seat. He sits down as far back into the chair as possible (Fig. 40).

(c) *One helper.* The above procedure is followed with the helper standing at the weaker side. The helper uses the palm-to-palm thumb grasp, also giving support under the arm with her forearm.

The helper's foot must be so placed as to prevent the handicapped person's foot from slipping, and her knee to "block" the knee.

8. Sitting to the floor

(a) *For a handicapped person with weakness down one side.* If help is necessary the helper stands behind and to the affected side; she may kneel with one knee on the bed or chair. She can assist either by placing her hands under the handicapped person's armpits or by holding and lifting from the waistband of the trousers or skirt.

The handicapped person turns towards his normal side and places his hand on the bed or chair (taking care not to tip the chair).

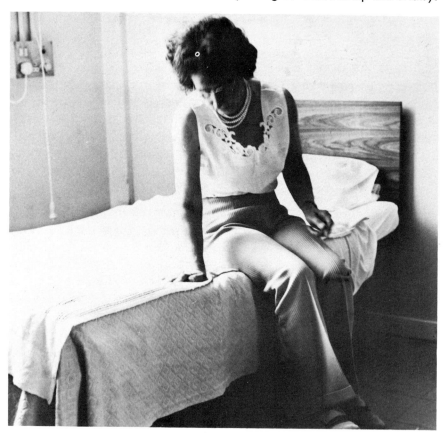

Fig. 41 (a). *From sitting to the floor for a person weak down one side:
starting position*

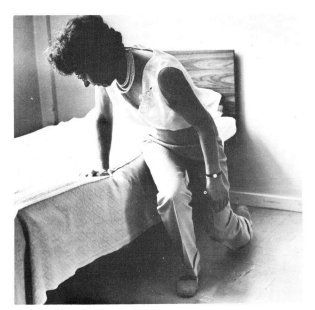

Fig. 41(b). *From sitting to the floor for a person weak down one side: turning to kneel*

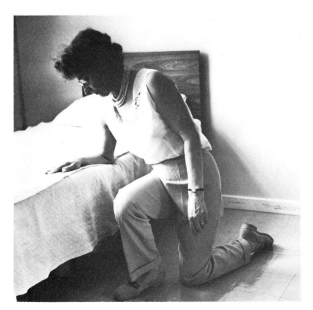

Fig. 41(c). *From sitting to the floor for a person weak down one side: kneeling and leaning*

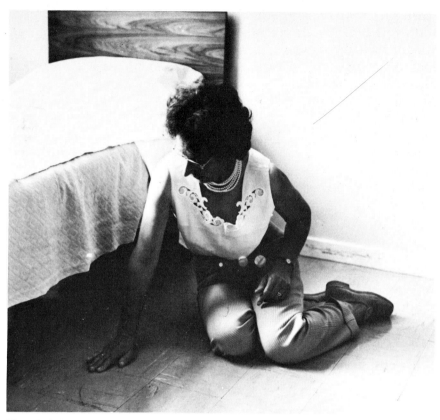

Fig. 41 (d).   *From sitting to the floor for a person weak down one side:
sitting on the hips and turning to one side*

He takes his weight on the normal hand and leg and raises his hips.
He then kneels on the knee of the weaker outer leg while the knee
of the normal leg remains at a right angle with the foot firmly on the
floor. Next he takes his weight on the normal hand and as far as
possible on the weaker knee and moves the normal leg into the
kneeling position (Figs. 41 (a)–(d)). From this position he can
either assume the all-fours position or turn to face the chair or bed
and sit down sideways towards the unaffected side.

(b) *For the handicapped person with little strength in his legs but
good power in his arms*

   (i) The above method can be modified but both the handicapped
person's hands must grasp and press on the seat, and he then

rotates further to one side. This should result in the knees bending further and descending a little towards the floor. By taking his weight fully on both hands the handicapped person can raise his hips off the seat. If the rotary movement is continued, he can lower himself carefully on to his knees. When the move is completed he is in the kneeling position facing the chair.

(ii) If the handicapped person is strong in the arms he can use the forward transfer method. He goes down in two stages from the chair to a solid cushion or foot-stool (Fig. 42(a)) and sits from foot-stool to floor (Fig. 42(b)). The handicapped person must lift his hips clear and avoid scraping his back on the chair or bed on the way down.

(c) *Assisted lowering of a handicapped person to the floor.*

(i) *The through-arm lift* (Fig. 22, p. 34). Two helpers work together, one at the head and the other at the legs. It is vital that the helpers keep their backs straight and lower the handicapped person to the sitting position by bending their hips and knees.

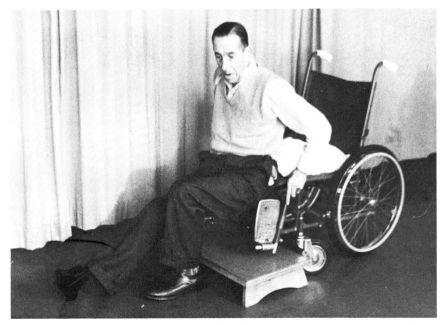

Fig. 42(a).　*Straight transfer to the floor for a person with strong arms from chair to foot-stool*

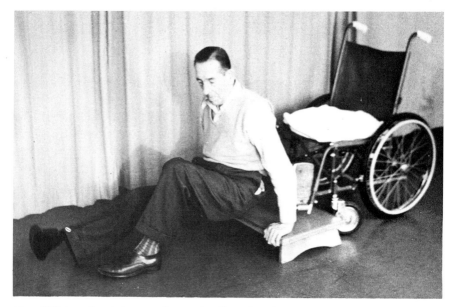

Fig. 42(b). *Straight transfer to the floor for a person with strong arms from foot-stool to floor*

(ii) *The through-arm lift using one helper.* If the handicapped person can stand, the helper can lower him safely to the floor (Fig. 43). The handicapped person must be held close to the helper's body. This method is not advised if the handicapped person is much taller than the helper.

(iii) *The shoulder lift.* It is possible to use this lift (Figs. 18(a) and (b), pp. 29, 30), although it is probably more difficult than the through-arm lift.

9. Floor to chair

The reverse of the methods advised in the section above may be used, except that two helpers may find the palm-to-palm thumb grasp is better than the through-arm grasp. The feet may need to be blocked.

10. Assisted walking

(a) *Basic hold.* The helper or helpers stand to the side. They use the palm-to-palm thumb grasp with the other hand round the upper arm or round the waist.

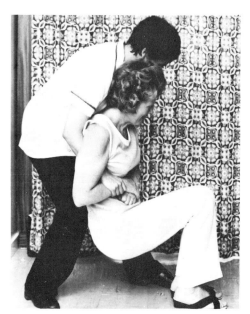

Fig. 43. *Through-arm lift by one helper from floor to standing*

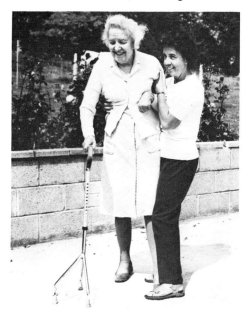

Fig. 44. *Assisted walking*

(b) *For a handicapped person with weakness down one side.* The helper stands at the weaker side and supports from behind with an arm round the waist. The other hand can support either from in front under the armpit or with the palm-to-palm thumb grasp. The forward leg of the helper is positioned to block the foot and support the weaker knee when weight is taken on it (Fig. 44). Generally the best walking pattern is stick forward, weaker leg forward, stronger leg forward, but occasionally people use stick forward, stronger leg forward, weaker leg forward.

By using the hand which is supporting at waist level, the helper can assist the handicapped person to change his weight from one foot to the other. It may be necessary for the helper to help the forward movement of the weaker leg with her own foot and knee from behind.

(c) *Assisted walking from behind.* This method is not generally used but may be useful on occasions. The helper needs to be at least as tall as the handicapped person. She stands behind him and places one of her hands between his arm and his body so that this hand can be placed firmly on the breast bone or shoulder.

The helper holds the handicapped person firmly between her hands and her own body, helping to keep him erect by pressure backward on the breast bone and forward on the bony area above the buttocks. She can assist him (i) to get weight over the standing leg by pushing him gently towards that side, or (ii) to move his legs forward by using his own leg, and if necessary the free front hand may be used to lift the leg or caliper through.

11. Axillary (underarm) crutches

The basic methods of using axillary crutches for a handicapped person able to stand on only one leg are indicated in this section. Unless the person has good balance a helper should be at hand.

It is very important that crutches are of the correct length. There must be no pressure under the armpit as important nerves and blood vessels would be subject to compression. Therefore the crutches must not be too long. If they are too short they can slip.

The weight must be taken on the hands and the padded underarm section pressed against the ribs, thus "propping" the body up on either side. The hand-pieces should be fixed so that the elbows are only slightly bent.

(a) *Standing from sitting*

(i) The principles of standing from sitting apply. Both the crutches are held in the hand of the affected side. The grip is as used for a stick (overgrip). The handicapped person stands by pushing on the crutches with the one hand and on the chair with the other. He then transfers one crutch to the other hand and rotates both crutches to the underarm position.

(ii) The very well-balanced and strong person may start with a crutch in each hand. The grip is again as for holding a stick. He stands using the crutches and thrusts with his leg. Having established balance, he rotates the crutches into the underarm position.

(b) *Sitting from standing.* The procedure for standing from sitting is reversed. The handicapped person must ensure that he is near to the seat before he sits.

(c) *Standing.* The crutches must be pressed against the ribs. To ensure good balance they must be angled a little outward and placed slightly in advance of the standing leg, giving a triangular base.

(d) *Walking*

(i) *Swing-to method.* This method is advisable for older people and others with poor balance and strength.

Weight is taken on the crutches through the hands. The elbows should straighten slightly. As the weight is taken off the main weight-bearing leg, the foot is lifted off the ground and brought forward to a point slightly behind the crutches.

If the older person were to find himself with his crutches behind his feet, it is possible that he would fall backward.

(ii) *Swing-through method.* This method is usually adopted by younger people with strong arms and shoulders and good balance.

The method is as above except that the foot is brought "through" in front of the crutches. This has to be a continuous movement with the walker's momentum taking him forward into the next sequence.

(e) *Up and down stairs*

(i) *Up.* The "good" leg is taken on to the step above. The crutches follow.

(ii) *Down.* The crutches are taken on to the step below. The leg follows.

The helper must always be between the handicapped person and the "drop" and ensure that the disabled leg is clear of the step.

12. Carrying a child
When carrying a handicapped child it may be very important to give adequate support to the head and back. The child is held closely. The helper places the child's arms over her shoulders and his legs round her waist. The helper supports the child's buttocks with one hand and his head and back with the other hand and arm (Fig. 45).

13. Wheelchair and stairs
(a) *One step or kerb.* This does not usually present any problems.

(i) A ramp may be fixed at any point where regular use is anticipated.

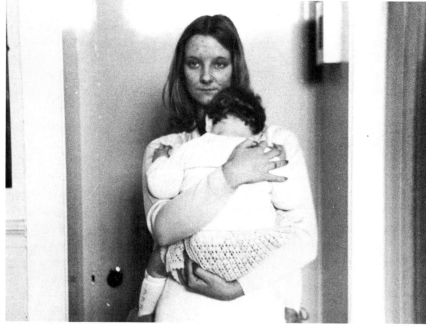

Fig. 45. *Carrying a child: the upper hand can, if necessary, be used to support the head*

(ii) A helper can easily negotiate a step by tipping the chair backward by pressing down on the handles and with one foot on the metal spokes provided and manoeuvring the chair on the larger back wheels.

(b) *A flight of stairs.* This is not an impossible barrier with two strong helpers. The helpers stand one at the back and the other at the front of the chair. The helper at the back grasps the handles and tips the chair backward. The helper at the front, facing forward (back to the person in the chair) keeping his back straight, crouches down and grasps the framework of the chair behind her. Care must be taken not to grasp any detachable or movable part of the chair. The helper at the front stands, tipping the person in the chair further on to his back. Both helpers take the strain and lift the chair and its occupant. It is very important for the chair to be tipped well back so that the handicapped person is facing the ceiling. Stairs can be negotiated with safety in this way. When coming down it may be convenient carefully to "bump" the chair down each step.

14. Emergency situations

(a) *Falls.* If a handicapped person falls, it is essential for the helpers to assess the extent of any injuries before attempting to move him.

If there is any doubt whatsoever as to the injuries sustained, the handicapped person must be made comfortable and kept warm, without changing his position, until expert help is available.

If the fall has occurred in a confined space, the handicapped person should be adjusted until he is secure in a sitting position. The through-arm lift may then be used. If the fall has occurred in an open space either the through-arm lift or shoulder lift may be used (*see* Chapter 3, pp. 22–35).

(b) *In the bath.* If an emergency occurs when a handicapped person is in the bath and he needs to be lifted rather than assisted out, it is unwise for one person to attempt this unaided. The water should be let out of the bath. This will make the lifting easier. The person in the bath should be dried and kept warm with towels and possibly a blanket. When a second helper has been found, a stool or chair is placed parallel with the bath at hip level, the through-arm lift should be used, and the most experienced lifter take the head and shoulders. The ordinary domestic bath is usually low and fitted so that one cannot get between the wall and the head of the bath. To avoid strain each lifter should place her near foot into the bath. A towel in the bath may give a better foothold, especially if a non-slip bath mat is not in place. The handicapped person can then be lifted on to the chair in one movement, or rested for a moment on the side of the bath to allow the helpers to adjust their positions.

Chapter 5

HOISTS AND BEDS

Veronica R. Adams, M.C.S.P.

When a person is unable to transfer with ease from his wheelchair to the bed, bath or W.C., great physical and mental strain is often put on other relatives with the constant fear that he may fall and be unable to get up again.

After all other methods of transfer have been tried and failed, the use of a mechanical hoist may be indicated. A disabled person can be supplied with a hoist by the Social Services Department of his own area, which will send a suitable member of staff to visit him. When a disabled person receives a hoist he is often able to achieve greater mobility, thus enabling him to perform some independent activity within the home. This device, without doubt, can help to relieve some of the frustration which often surrounds a disabled person who is dependent on others.

Selecting a Hoist

It is very important that the person who is to be assessed for a hoist is assessed by a competent therapist because this type of equipment is expensive. It is preferable that both he and his relatives should try out the system before any costly home installation is embarked upon. This can be done in several ways:

1. Referral of the handicapped person to a specialised assessment centre by the G.P. or hospital consultant.
2. A visit to the Disabled Living Foundation Information Centre. This is a permanent exhibition staffed by occupational therapists (the public can visit by appointment only). Here people can try out various hoists and obtain advice.
3. A visit with a therapist to the home of someone who already possesses a hoist to enable the disabled person and relatives to try it out.

Before obtaining a hoist the relatives must be sure that they have been recommended the correct type by a therapist and that they know how to operate it and can cope with the various types of slings. There must be adequate space to manoeuvre the hoist in the home and there should be enough storage space.

Some points to be considered when selecting a hoist are the age and disability of the patient, the age and fitness of the operator, the purpose for which the hoist is to be used, the size of the area in which it is to be manoeuvred, and the available storage space.

Main Types of Hoist

Types of hoist can be divided into two main categories: electric hoists which can often be self-operated; and portable hoists which are always attendant-operated. Bath and car hoists will be considered later.

1. Electric hoists
These are mains-operated hoists which are attached to a ceiling track or to an overhead gantry (Fig. 46). It may be possible for a

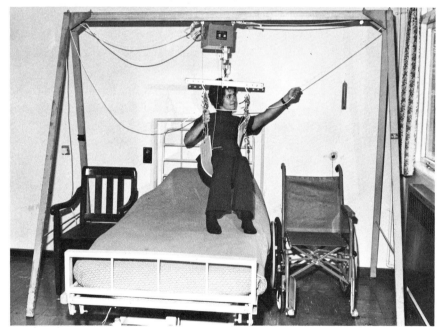

Wessex Medical Equipment Co.
Fig. 46. *Wessex electric hoist with gantry frame*

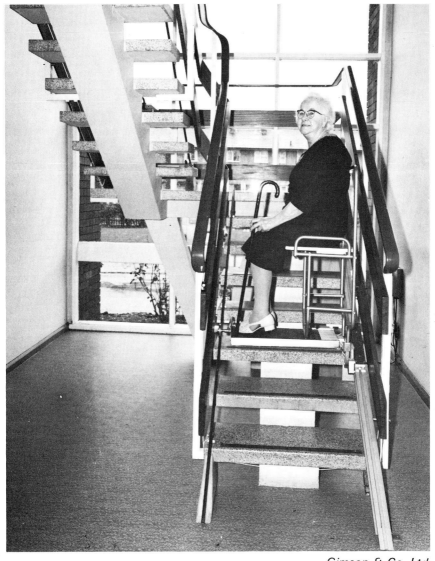

Gimson & Co. Ltd.

Fig. 47. *Stairider unit*

continuous ceiling track to be fixed between the bedroom and bathroom, so allowing transfers to bed, W.C. and bath using only one hoist box. This means that the structural layout of the house needs careful attention. Alternatively, two ceiling tracks can be installed, and a light type of hoist box such as a Commodore Minor can be transferred from one track to the other. The advantage of the overhead tracking system is that the floor space is left clear, an important consideration in today's small houses.

When considering a ceiling attachment it is essential to obtain advice from a builder to check that the joists are strong enough to hold the track and the person. In the case of local authority housing a check should also be made with the local council to obtain permission for a permanent fixture.

An alternative is the use of a portable gantry frame. This can be obtained in a variety of lengths to suit the person's needs and the size of the room in which it is to stand; e.g. if the person requires a single bed, wheelchair and commode to stand together under the hoist, ideally he would require a 9-ft gantry.

The operation of an electric hoist requires little physical strength. The up–down mechanism is operated by a light pull on one of two coloured ropes; this often allows a person with weak muscle power in the hands to operate it without difficulty, even though he may be unable to position the slings. Movement in a horizontal plane is slightly more difficult but may be done by pulling another rope through a system of pulleys.

This type of hoist can also be used for transferring a patient up a flight of stairs or through a trapdoor from one floor to another. Here again, builders would need to be contacted to ensure the feasibility of the idea.

The problem of mounting a flight of stairs could also be overcome by using a stairlift; the "Stairider" is a self-contained unit which is suitable for fixing to any straight stairway. The standard unit is fitted with a hinged platform which can be used to support a wheelchair and occupant. An alternative is a folding seat which can be attached to the lift if required (Fig. 47).

The carrying capacity of this type of lift is 250 lb, and it is fitted with a positive safety device which immediately arrests the platform in the event of a mechanical failure. "Call" and "send" push-buttons are installed at the top and bottom of the stairs.

2. Portable hoists

The advantage of a portable hoist is that it can be used for transferring the disabled person in different rooms. It can be used by a

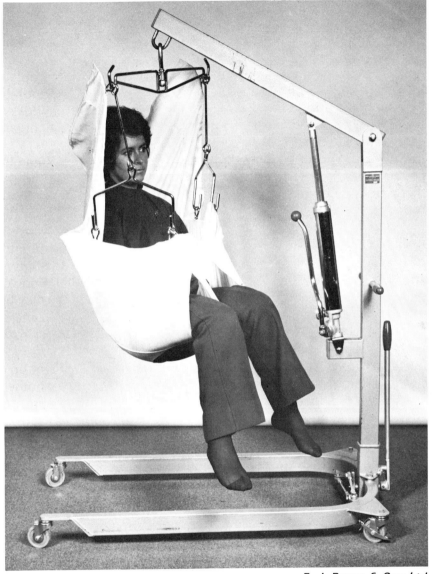

Fig. 48. *New Oxford Hoist using a hammock sling*

reasonably fit relative to transfer a person from the bed to bath or
W.C. with minimal physical effort. These hoists can also be used to
transfer some people in or out of a car. But before any relative

obtains such a hoist it is important that he should be shown how to operate it properly.

A variety of portable hoists can be issued by local authorities. Some examples are as follows:

(a) *New Oxford Hoist* (Fig. 48). This is a pneumatic hoist operated by a pumping action to raise the patient and by a release valve to lower him. The rate of descent is controlled by the amount the valve is opened. To ensure that the person is seated well on to the chair the knees should be pushed well back towards the seat of the chair by the operator. This hoist is now made with a low chassis (height 4 in.) so that clearance under a car or bed should not present any problem.

The legs of the hoist are adjustable in width to allow easy access to wide armchairs and wheelchairs. The brakes on the castors must be applied to allow complete stability before hoisting is begun.

(b) *Mecalift* (Fig. 49). This is a small, manoeuvrable type of portable hoist operated by winding a handle. The hoist can be fitted with a wide chassis to accommodate wide chairs, and a height extension is now available which allows easier access to higher beds and baths. The hoist can be taken apart for storage and can be packed into the boot of some cars.

Operation of both these hoists is facilitated by a smooth floor covering and hindered by rough carpets and rugs. Obviously, steps between one room and another present a problem. Sometimes these can be ramped by the local authority.

Other Types of Hoist

1. Car hoists

If the use of a portable hoist for car transfers is impracticable, a car hoist may be the answer. These are operated either hydraulically or electrically from the car battery. Both types of hoist require an attendant to operate them.

The hoist is attached to the roof of the car by means of suction feet and clamps. The boom telescopes into the frame and the lifting arm folds up to rest in a clip for travelling (Figs. 50 and 51). Standard slings can be used with these hoists; frequently the chains have to be short to allow easier entry into the car.

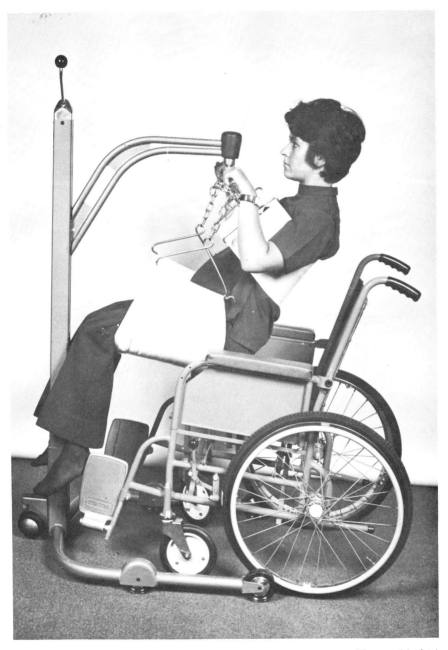

Fig. 49. *Mecalift using two band slings*

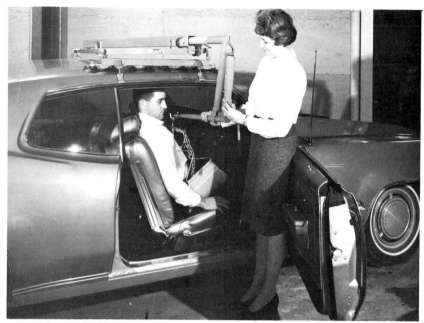

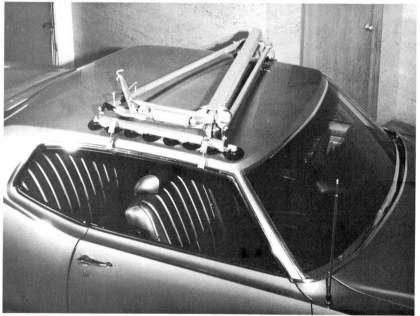

Fig. 50.   *Hoyer Kartop hoist*

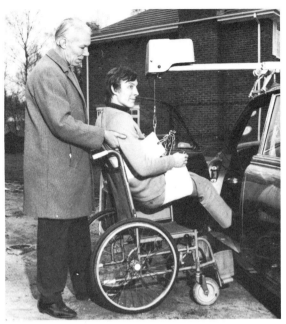

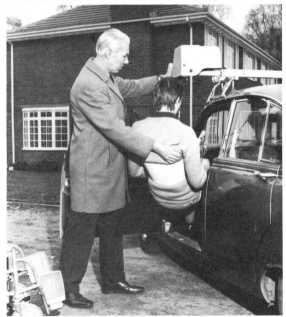

S. Burvill & Son

Fig. 51. Burvill car hoist

Manufacturers of these hoists will often arrange a home demonstration so that a person may try out the hoist on his own car. Car hoists usually have to be bought privately, but sometimes a local authority will supply them if the disabled person can show a need for travelling to his place of work.

2. Bath hoists

An electric hoist with an overhead track, as previously described, can be fixed in a bathroom to allow transfers from wheelchair to bath and W.C. The electrical supply to the hoist is by means of an isolating transformer which provides the low voltage to comply

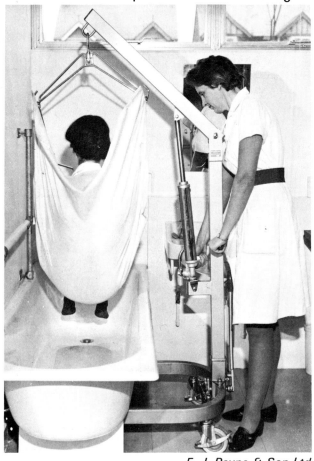

F. J. Payne & Son Ltd.

Fig. 52.   *New Oxford hoist used for the bath*

with the safety requirements of the Institute of Electrical Engineers *Regulations for Electrical Equipment for Buildings.*

If the handicapped person requires a portable hoist it may be necessary to cut out a small length of boarding in the side panel of the bath in order to allow the chassis of the hoist to be pushed underneath. In some cases the bath itself may have to be raised (Fig. 52).

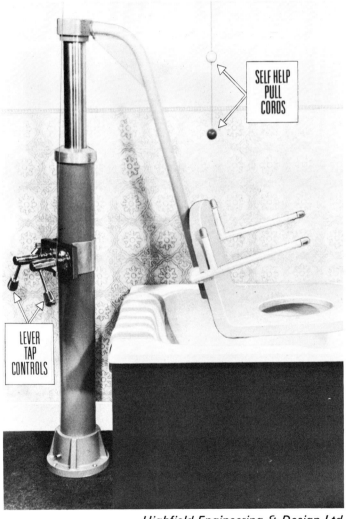

SELF HELP
PULL
CORDS

LEVER
TAP
CONTROLS

Highfield Engineering & Design Ltd.
Fig. 53.   *Spa bath lift*

Alternatively, the New Oxford Hoist boom and mast can be sunk into a turntable fixed into the bathroom floor. The person can then be swung round from the wheelchair to the bath. This allows easy bath transfers in an area where space is often at a premium. Again, a builder's advice should be sought as to whether the particular floor would be suitable for this arrangement.

There is also now a bath hoist which is similarly fixed to the floor but which can be self-operated, an advantage people may often prefer (Fig. 53).

Slings

When using a hoist it is important to find the correct type of sling to give maximum comfort and safety to the person concerned. Often a handicapped person needs a different arrangement of slings for different activities.

The slings can be made of a variety of materials such as nylon, canvas or Covertex. A washable sling is an obvious advantage as most would be used for bathing or toilet purposes. Examples of common slings are as follows:

1. *Band slings* are suitable for less disabled people with reasonable postural control. Two separated band slings are used (Fig. 49), a narrow one placed behind the handicapped person's back and a wider one placed under his thighs or vice versa as preferred. These are the easiest type to position under the person and can sometimes be inserted by the person being hoisted. The slings are then attached by chains on to the spreader bar of the hoist.

2. *A one-piece hammock sling* extends from the head or upper trunk right through to the thighs (*see* Fig. 48).

Use of a hammock sling is indicated for the more disabled person, often with a lack of head control and weak postural muscles. If the person has upper limb pain or general joint pain, the hammock sling gives more support and allows less joint movement than the band slings.

The inside thigh-pieces of the sling may be crossed over to prevent the legs swinging out. On the other hand, for toilet purposes, it may be easier to leave the thigh-pieces uncrossed. If removal of the split-leg hammock sling is difficult the person can remain sitting on it during the day. This allows a less time-consuming manoeuvre when the chains and spreader bar are attached.

3. *Other types of hammock sling* are made with a toilet aperture in the seat. The person must be rolled on to this type of sling in bed and then remain on it all day. Adaptations can be made to all hammock slings for individual problems.

4. *Harness sling* (Fig. 54). If a person with general muscle weakness, *e.g.* muscular dystrophy, has difficulty in rising from the

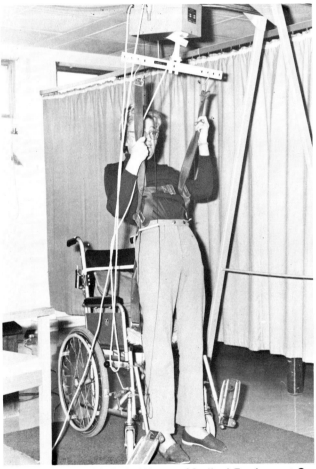

Railvalift Ltd.; Wessex Medical Equipment Co.

Fig. 54.   *A Railvalift harness sling in use with a Wessex hoist*

floor or a chair, a parachute harness may sometimes allow him to do this independently. This type of harness has been found successful by many people who have been worried by the fear of falling and being unable to get up again if they are alone. Because these patients present a difficult problem, expert advice should be sought.

Beds

When considering the transfer of a disabled person from one place to another, it is sensible to consider the type of bed. Although the bed may need to be high for nursing purposes, the disabled person may experience difficulty in arising. The answer may be an adjustable bed such as a King's Fund bed (Fig. 55). This is a hard-based bed raised and lowered by a pedal. It can be elevated at the foot into positions suitable for leg elevation, or for drainage of the lungs if the person has a chest problem.

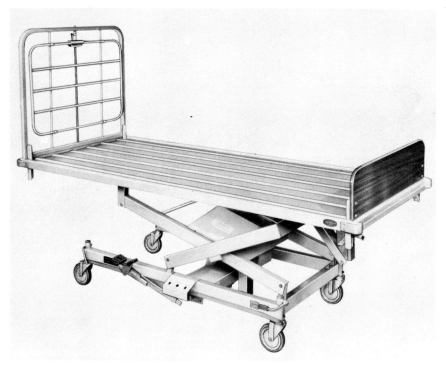

J. Nesbit-Evans & Co. Ltd.
Fig. 55.   *King's Fund bed Mark III*

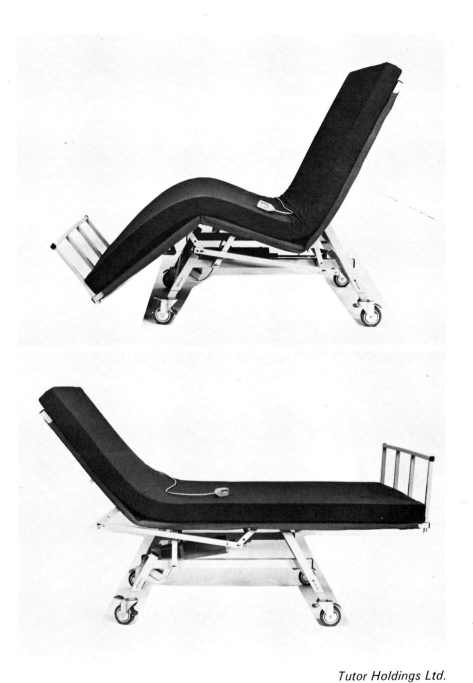

Fig. 56.   *Tutormatic electric bed*

Relatives may find an electrically operated bed of benefit for moving unaided a heavy person from a lying to a sitting position (Figs. 56, 57 and 58). The beds are operated by a press-button switch which slowly raises and lowers the back-rest.

Some beds are adjustable to a chair position, which is very helpful for bedridden persons who really do require a change of position during the day or night.

A waterbed (Fig. 59) provides a mattress that helps the healing of pressure sores. It can also be used as a prophylactic measure to prevent development of sores in handicapped people. People with bent knees and hips often find this surface much more tolerable than an ordinary mattress. The warmth of the water also aids muscular relaxation. The mattress rests in a glass fibre container which is mounted on a polystyrene base. A specially shaped base can be supplied if there is need for a hoist to be placed underneath.

Adjustable heating to maintain a constant temperature of the water is provided by a specially built-in system that is completely sealed within the base of the frame. The recommended temperature for use is 30°C to 32°C. The mattress can be filled with water from a garden hose.

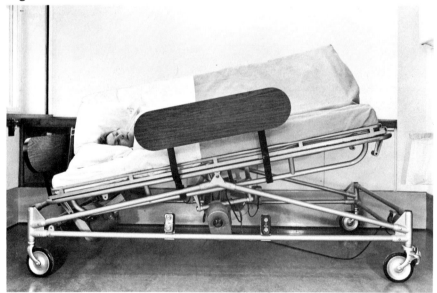

Egerton Hospital Equipment Ltd.
Fig. 57.   *Egerton tilting and turning bed*

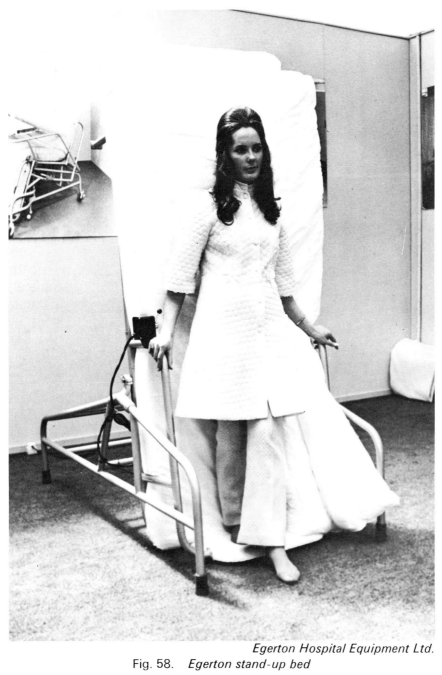

Egerton Hospital Equipment Ltd.

Fig. 58.   Egerton stand-up bed

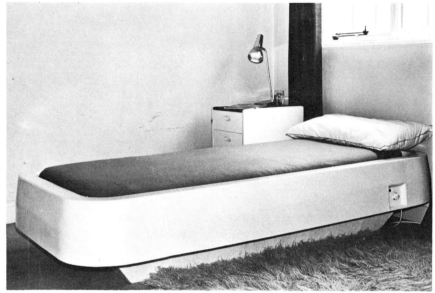

Fig. 59.   *Aquadorm waterbed*

Summary

Handicapped people can be helped in many ways by being supplied with aids such as hoists and special beds. It is important to realise that, where more than one aid is required, compatibility between them must be achieved. Handicapped people can be taught to lead a much more independent way of life provided they have been given the correct pieces of equipment. Hoists and beds are expensive and it is important for both the person and relatives to work out what is required and consult their local authority. Several charities for the disabled also may be willing to contribute towards the cost of this equipment.

A list of addresses of manufacturers of hoists and beds is given at the end of the book.

Chapter 6

WHEELCHAIRS

J. Tanner, M.B.A.O.T.

A wheelchair can vary from a simple means of transport used on an occasional outing to a handicapped person's sole means of independent mobility. Many types are available and if one is to be used permanently it is essential to choose the right model. Experienced medical and technical help is needed to make this selection, and therefore wheelchairs are described here only briefly: more important are the details of how to obtain and use one, and where to seek help.

Types of Wheelchair

The choice of chair will vary with the patient's disability, where and when he will use it, and where it is to be stored. Sometimes more than one chair is needed for different purposes. Discussion with a doctor is essential.

1. *Self-propelling, folding chairs*, with large wheels at the back (Fig. 60), are the most common, although a model with large self-propelling wheels at the front (Fig. 61) is very manoeuvrable and useful for people with limited shoulder movement. Large front wheels do, however, impede sideways transfers and make a close approach to a bed or cupboards very difficult. They can also make movement outside difficult as kerbs cannot be negotiated; nor can an attendant tip the chair to surmount obstacles.
2. *Non-folding or rigid chairs* are often upholstered and some are also available with commode facilities. They can be very manoeuvrable, but all rigid chairs are large and rather cumbersome, and adequate room for storage is essential.
3. *Car transit chairs* (Fig. 62) have either two 12-in. back wheels and front swivel castors or four fixed 12-in. wheels. This does not mean, however, that they cannot be self-propelled and many people use their feet to kick themselves along or use two sticks to "punt"

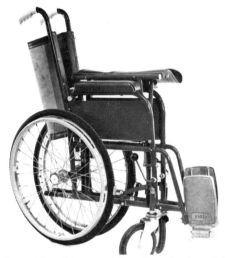

Fig. 60. *Vessa 8G. Standard adult heavy-duty chair. It can be self propelled. The foot-rests, however, are normally fixed*

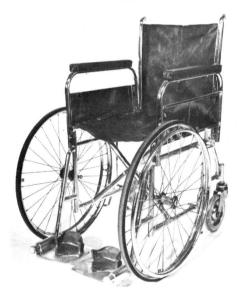

Fig. 61. *Everest & Jennings Front-Wheel Drive. Large wheels at the front make propelling easier for those with stiff shoulders*

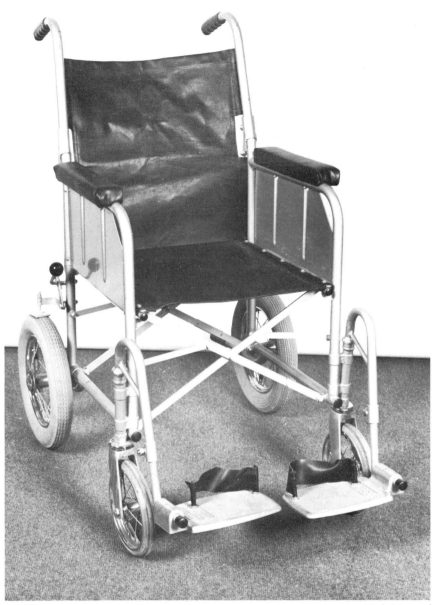

Fig. 62. *Bencraft 9L. This chair is light and useful for car use as it folds and has a folding back-rest also*

very successfully (Fig. 63). All fold and the majority have hinged back-rests making them compact when folded and easy to stow in a car boot (Fig. 64). Many wheelchair riders like the four pneumatic tyres offered by some of these chairs, but many attendants find them extremely difficult to manage as they must be tipped or lifted like a pram each time a corner is turned. If this is the case, a chair fitted with swivel castors is usually chosen and these are essential for those propelling themselves.

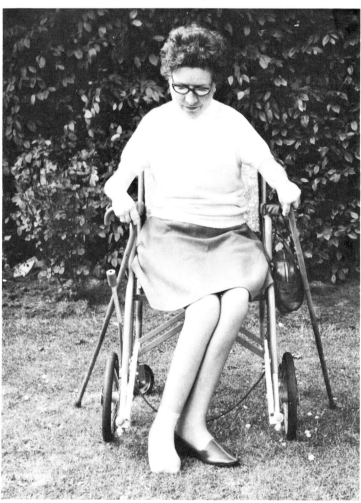

Fig. 63.   *A special car transit. A car transit chair being propelled by two sticks,* i.e. *"punted"*

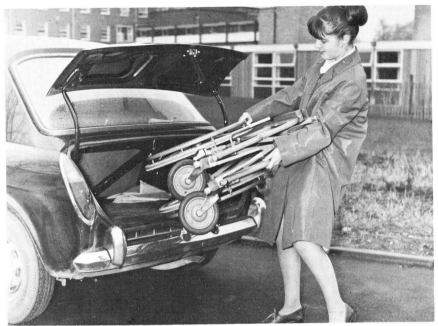

Fig. 64.   *Lifting a wheelchair into the boot of a car*

4. *Outdoor chairs*. Most chairs already described can be used either indoors or out. Specifically outdoor models are sprung and upholstered and have a weather apron (Fig. 65). They are designed to be pushed by an attendant and are comfortable during long, rough journeys. Although they fold, they are not so compact as the car transit chair and storage in a car or house may be difficult.

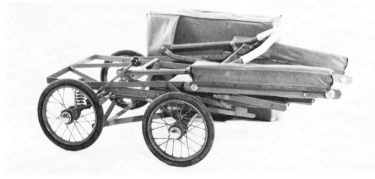

Fig. 65.   *Tan Sad Model 13. These comfortable outdoor models do fold but are heavy and need adequate storage space*

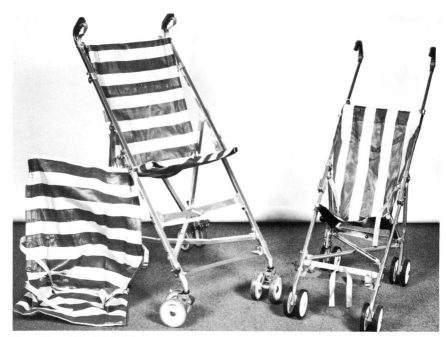

Fig. 66. *Model 21 (Buggy Major) and Model 21C (Baby Buggy). On the right is the Baby Buggy and left the Buggy Major, which can be fitted with an intermediate insert if necessary. These two Andrews MacLaren models then provide three progressive seat sizes. All are lightweight and fold easily*

5. *Lightweight chairs* (weighing about 30 lb) are a boon for the not-so-strong. However, standard weight chairs (weighing approximately 50 lb and upwards) are robust and essential for continual or heavy adult use and can also be made in outsize models. All chairs are lighter to lift, whether up steps or into a car boot, if foot-pieces, arm-rests, cushions, trays and so on are removed first.
6. *Children's chairs.* There is a special range of chairs for children. The first a baby might have is a Baby Buggy (Fig. 66, *right*), a lightweight pushchair easily folded and carried on public transport. The larger version of this (Fig. 66, *centre*) is equally lightweight and convenient. It has an insert (Fig. 66, *left*) which provides an intermediate-sized seat. Both these chairs, however, are not strong enough for rough wear and, although ideal for city pavements and indoor use, will not withstand continual use over rough ground. The trolley shown in Fig. 67 (*right*) may be a youngster's first

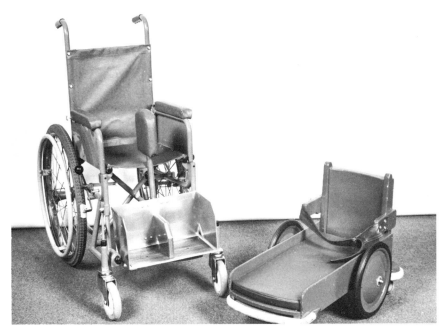

Fig. 67.   *Vessa 8C and Chailey Chariot. The "chariot"* (right) *may be a child's first self-propelling chair. The large one* (left) *is robust and stable and can have several accessories fitted*

self-propelling "chair". It allows him to move freely at floor level and has a safety strap and cushion to protect sensitive skin. Once a child is older, the chair shown in Fig. 67 (*left*) may be chosen. Again the youngster can push himself, and this particular model provides a very stable, robust chair that will withstand rough playground use. It is shown fitted with an optional footbox and a pommel, and other modifications can be included.

7. *Special chairs for individual requirements.* One such chair is a single-arm control chair (Fig. 68), for those who have the use of only one hand. It can, however, be difficult to control for those who find learning hard and it is often found that the "one hand, one foot" method is more satisfactory in a standard model. Perseverance with the latter method usually brings satisfaction.

Another more specialised chair is the fully reclining chair made by Everest & Jennings. (Fig. 75, p. 102). The back- and foot-rests can be adjusted to the horizontal position and to many stages in between. A semi-recliner reclines to a 30° angle. Difficulties can

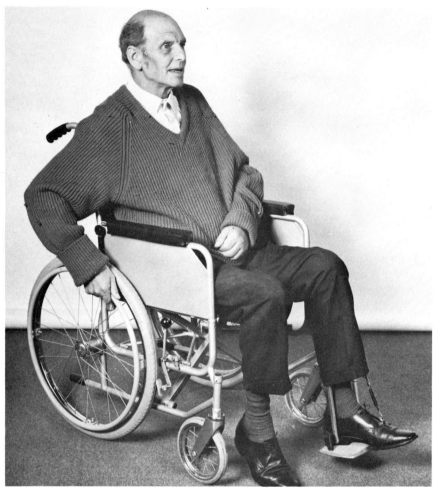

Fig. 68. *Bencraft 8L. Standard chairs can be propelled with practice using the "one hand, one foot" method. They are often easier to manage than the more complicated "one-handed" models*

arise from the upright rod of the reclining mechanism as it can obstruct a person transferring sideways.

Perhaps the smallest of all adult chairs is the Everest & Jennings Glideabout (Fig. 69). This is virtually a "kitchen chair" on castors and is only 20 in. wide. Made with or without arms, brakes or foot-rests, it is pushed with the feet. For some whose walking balance is poor it can be very useful.

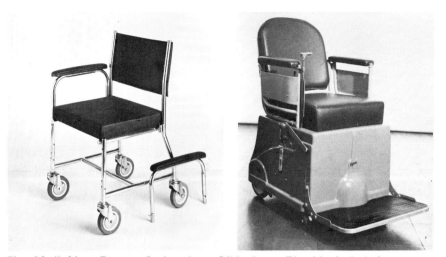

Fig. 69 (left). *Everest & Jennings Glideabout. The ideal chair for narrow spaces and small rooms. It is a pushchair only, however, or needs to be propelled by foot*

Fig. 70 (right). *A.C. Epic 102. One of the smallest powered indoor chairs. It is easy to drive and turns in small areas. It cannot, however, be free-wheeled*

8. *Powered chairs*. Some people who are unable to move about in an ordinary wheelchair may be eligible for a powered model. Again there are many different sorts. The A.C. Epic (Fig. 70) is perhaps the smallest and most easily managed and has an upholstered back and seat. Unfortunately it does not fold and cannot be pushed when not under power—two possible drawbacks. The chairs made by Everest & Jennings (one model is shown in Fig. 71) and by the B.E.C. Company all fold and have the added advantage of coming in either junior or adult sizes. Powered chairs tend to be large and need varying degrees of turning space, so that the user's housing must be considered. Some will take rough ground and ramps in house or garden, while others will cope only with smooth, level areas. All electric chairs come with the equipment necessary for charging and with directions for simple maintenance. In the street they may be used only on pavements because they have no emergency braking facilities and are not licensed as powered vehicles. One outdoor powered model is available through the Department of Health and Social Security but this is an attendant-controlled model—it may be supplied if the handicapped person is

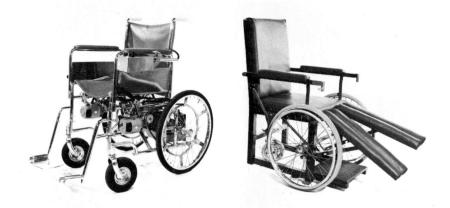

Fig. 71 (left). *Everest & Jennings Powerdrive. A more robust powered indoor chair that can be used to a limited extent outside. Available in junior and adult models and can be pushed by an attendant if the battery runs out*

Fig. 72 (right). *Model I with elevating leg-rests. Trays and many types of elevating leg-rests can be fitted to chairs. This particular indoor model may also have a commode fitting*

normally pushed by a helper who has now become infirm or if he lives in a hilly district.

Both special and powered chairs require the advice of a consultant. The G.P. will refer a handicapped person to a local Wheelchair Clinic at a hospital or an Artificial Limb and Appliance Centre (A.L.A.C.).

Optional Extras

There are dozens of additional fittings which can adapt a wheelchair for individual users.

1. *Trays* are available to fit almost all chairs and those with removable arm-rests normally have sockets into which the tray slips (Fig. 72). The arm-rests are simply reversed so that the bungs are at the front, making sure the side cover remains to the outside (transposing to the right and left rests) or the chair seat will be narrower with the covers inside and may become uncomfortable. Other fittings are also available.

2. *Cushions* are available in many shapes and sizes. A paraplegic cushion shaped to take a urinal (Fig. 73) is invaluable for many.

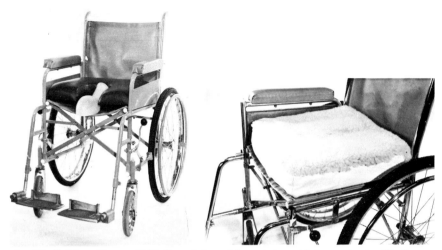

Fig. 73 (left).   *Vessa 8LV. Special cushions into which a urinal will slip are available for almost all chairs*

Fig. 74 (right).   *Cushions can be covered in sheepskin giving extra comfort and more protection for pressure-prone areas*

Sheepskin-covered cushions (Fig. 74) and battery-operated ripple cushions are also available and many find these particularly comfortable and useful in preventing pressure sores.

3. *Safety straps* are available in many forms. Straps are also available to support the heels, toes and legs.

4. *Head-rest extensions* may be fitted if the back of the chair is too low or the patient's head needs more support.

5. *Leg-rests and foot-rests.* Some chairs (Fig. 75) have fixed foot-rests and, although the foot-plates will swing up, the actual framework of the foot-rest does not alter. If an elevating leg-rest is needed, a bolt-on type may be obtained which although not recommended for permanent use is perfectly adequate for short-term use. The lightweight, self-propelling and car transit models have standard swinging detachable foot-rests. Elevating leg-rests are available for these and fit easily into the existing foot-rest sockets.

6. *Arm-rests.* Many chairs are fitted with detachable arm-rests. Some have a safety catch fitted. Figure 76 shows cutaway arms to allow access to desk or working surfaces.

7. *Capstans* (Fig. 77) are available for all self-propelling chairs.

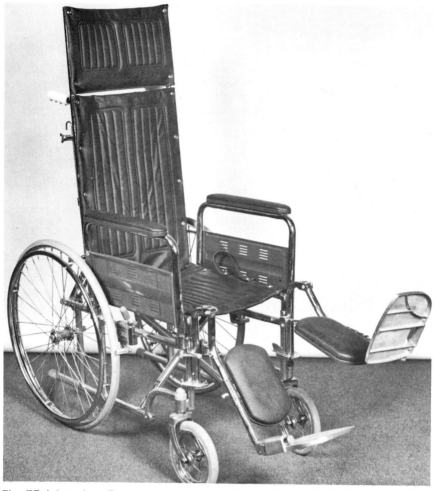

Fig. 75 (above).   *Everest & Jennings Fully Reclining Chair. This large chair is useful for those who need a reclining back-rest. Leg-rests are elevating and head-rest extensions can be fitted*

Fig. 76 (opposite, top).   *Everest & Jennings Single Arm Control Chair. Some who have the use of only one hand may find this chair an asset as it can be controlled from just one side. Many, however, find the "one hand, one foot" method easier (see Fig. 68). An extended brake lever and desk arms have also been fitted. Both are available on other models*

Fig. 77 (opposite, bottom).   *Everest & Jennings Adult Self Propelling Chair. Capstan hand rims can be fitted to all self-propelling models. They make it easier for those who, owing to weak grip, find propulsion difficult*

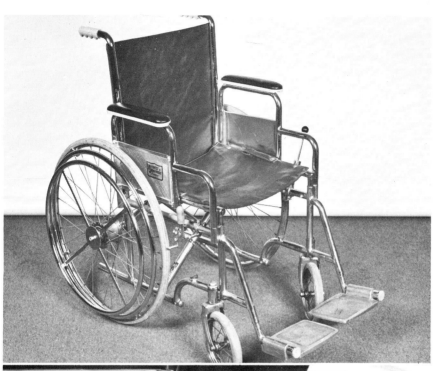

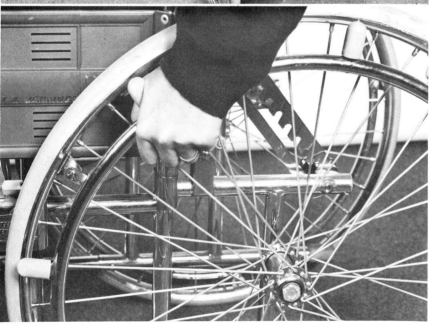

They allow a patient with poor hand function to control the propelling wheels more easily.

8. *Extended brake levers* may be built-in on many chairs or a slip-on extension can be fitted. This helps those who cannot reach the shorter brake and is easier for people with weak arms.

9. *Folding back-rests* are a boon in cars as the chair will fold smaller. They cannot be fitted to existing chairs, but many different makes and models can be obtained with such a device. They are not recommended for those who rely heavily on the back-rest for support or who suffer from severe back spasms. This is because the back-rest is slightly weakened at the join and, although perfectly safe for normal use, may wear quickly with continual heavy strain.

10. *Zip-back chairs* are invaluable in certain circumstances because the user can move or be moved backward out of the chair.

11. *Slope aids*. Several types of slope aids are available and some suit one person more than another. These prevent the chair from slipping backward when the rim is released to grasp it again.

12. *Ball-bearing arm supports* work on the principle that if gravity is counterbalanced and the weak arm well supported, the arm is able to move freely with very little muscle effort needed. They allow many people to use their hands to write, type, turn the pages of a book or feed themselves. They are, however, specialised aids which are not suitable for everyone. Expert medical advice is called for, firstly to assess whether they will be of benefit and secondly to fit them. A G.P. should be able to advise where this assessment can be done.

Cost of Wheelchairs

For people considered in need of a chair there is no charge. A suitable model will be provided by the Department of Health and Social Security. They may also be bought privately and a list of useful addresses is given at the end of the book.

Wheelchairs, particularly powered models, are very expensive and it is strongly recommended that the handicapped person should insist on a demonstration if possible in his own home, and personally try the chair before purchasing. If the chair belongs to the patient, he will have to pay for all repairs and spare parts. It may, however, be taken over by the D.H.S.S. which will then finance repairs for people considered eligible and prepared to accept any restrictions that may be imposed on its use. A G.P. can request State maintenance from the local A.L.A.C.

Some people may wish to obtain a chair for which they are not eligible under the N.H.S., such as a powered outdoor model or second indoor powered chair. Certain societies and benevolent funds which may help to finance this include the Armed Forces benevolent funds; professional and trade benevolent societies, such as the Musicians, Gardeners or Surveyors Benevolent Funds; and specific medical societies, such as the Multiple Sclerosis Society, Spastics Society, and Polio Fellowship. The local Social Services Department should be contacted for further details.

Hiring a Chair

Possible sources for the loan of a wheelchair are the Red Cross, the local authority, or the W.R.V.S. Any G.P. should be able to advise.

Repairs

The A.L.A.C. appoints official repairers and will supply the name of one to be contacted. With a minor problem such as a puncture a local garage or cycle shop may help. The bill can be sent to the local A.L.A.C. which will reimburse the handicapped person, but only up to a fixed limit, and so a preliminary inquiry is wise. A pump for pneumatic tyres is not automatically supplied with D.H.S.S. chairs, but one will be provided on request.

House Alterations

The local authority Social Services Department will send a qualified person to advise on ramps to cover steps, if it is possible to widen doors, and on any other structural difficulties in the home.

Help with a Car

People who need personal transport to and from a place of full-time work may be helped by being given a three- or (occasionally) four-wheeled car or a private car allowance. Details are available

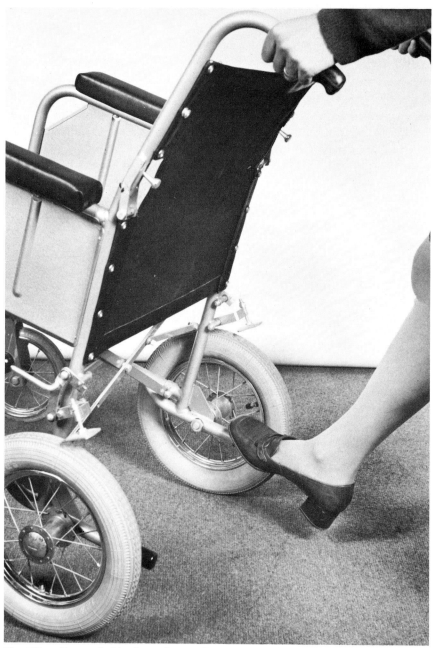

Fig. 78.   *Bencraft 9L. Attendants please note! Always use the tipping levers when turning a chair or surmounting an obstacle*

from the local A.L.A.C. or from the N.H.S. Leaflet 5, obtainable from the D.H.S.S. offices and local authority Social Services Departments. Users must be referred for consideration by a doctor.

Hints on Handling

1. Always use the tipping levers to turn a wheelchair (Fig. 78).

2. Make sure the covers of the arm-rests are on the outside.

3. Fold by adjusting the foot-plates upright and pulling the seat canvas up by the centre.

4. Open a chair by pressing down with both hands on the side tubes of the seat. Do not put fingers down the side of the chair!

5. If hands get dirty through propelling, make some palm mitts. Similarly plastic cuffs may protect sleeves.

6. Always remove leg- and arm-rests, cushions, trays and so on before lifting.

7. Lift a chair into a car boot by holding the frame as high as possible with one hand and as low down as possible with the other (Fig. 64, p. 95).

8. Always go up steps or the kerb with the large wheels first. Tip a patient back on to large wheels when going down.

9. Check front castors frequently for cotton and fluff.

10. If the chair is hard to push or propel, the tyres may be flat.

11. If sitting in the chair causes soreness, the foot-plates may be too high; they can easily be adjusted with a spanner. The thighs should be well supported and not too high. Alternatively a sheepskin or ripple cushion may help.

12. If the feet slip off the foot-plates, toe- or heel-loops may help.

Chapter 7

HANDLING IN THE SWIMMING POOL AREA

E. C. Trussell, J.P., M.C.S.P.
P. J. Waddington, M.C.S.P., Dip.T.P.

Methods of helping a handicapped swimmer before he reaches the pool—transfer from car to wheelchair, wheelchair to bench, bench to wheelchair and wheelchair to pool surround, for example—are the same as in any other circumstances and have been covered in previous chapters.

Before the swimmer is assisted into the water there must always be helpers both in the water and on the side of the pool. A wet towel or rubber mat should be placed over the edge of the pool to protect swimmers from hurting themselves on the side.

Into the Pool

1. Down a flight of steps or vertical ladder
(a) *Steps*. A helper should walk down in front of the swimmer.
(b) *Ladder.* A helper should stand in the water and guide and support the swimmer's legs and feet. Many swimmers who can manage steps may find a ladder too difficult.

2. Over the side of the pool
(a) The helper stands in the water and the swimmer sits over the side of the pool with his feet in the water. He leans forward and places his hands on the shoulders of the helper standing in the water. The helper grasps him round the waist and assists him into the pool. A second helper may be needed on the side (Fig. 79).

(b) The through-arm lift may be used to lift a sitting swimmer over the side of the pool. The helper on the side should ensure she does not injure her back. Again the swimmer is received into the pool by a second helper who takes care of his legs.

(c) Many swimmers can roll into the water from a lying position or "dive" into the pool from a sitting position. Care must be taken to ensure that they clear the rails and scum troughs round the inside edge of the pool.

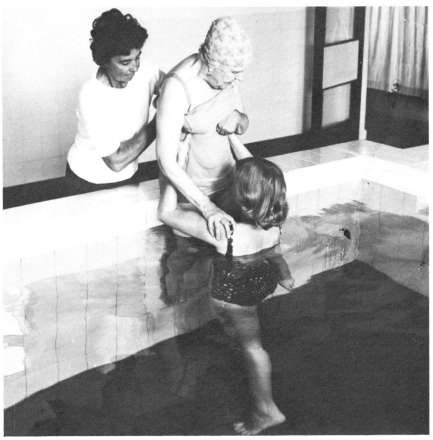

Fig. 79.   *The swimmer is helped from a sitting position on the side of the pool into the water, with one helper in and one out of the pool*

(d) Swimmers are occasionally lowered on a chair. A plain wooden chair may be used and basic rules of lifting must be applied. Three people may be needed to lift the swimmer and chair; the swimmer must be received by other helpers in the pool.

Out of the Pool

1. Up a flight of steps or vertical ladder
The helper should be behind the swimmer to guide his feet on to the steps and to ensure that they do not drag or, on a ladder, get caught between the rungs and the wall.

2. For the swimmer with two good arms but no power in his legs

Two helpers in the water at the shallow end stand on either side of the swimmer who has his back to the side of the pool. They get down in the water as low as possible by bending at the hips and knees, steadying themselves against the wall. They each get the shoulder nearer to the swimmer under his thigh and set him on their shoulders.

The swimmer places his hands on the edge of the pool.

Together, the swimmer thrusts with his arms and the helpers thrust with their hips, and the swimmer is hoisted into a sitting position on the side of the pool (Fig. 80).

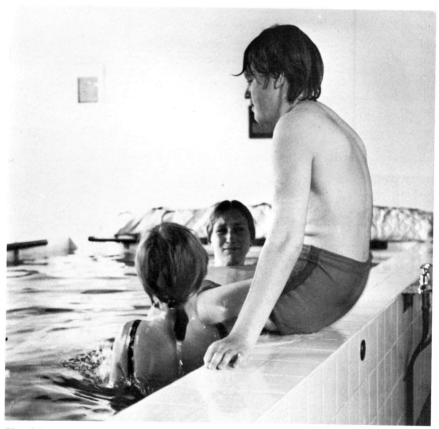

Fig. 80.   *The swimmer has been hoisted out of the pool to a sitting position on the side*

3. The bouncing method

This is much easier if the water level is raised. The side of the pool should be padded. The handicapped person is placed in the floating position parallel with the side of the pool with his arms folded across his body. He is advised not to attempt to help himself in any way.

The helpers face the side of the pool and place their straight arms, palms down, under the handicapped person's body. The helper at the head end places one arm under the shoulders and if necessary controls the head; her second arm is placed at waist level. The helper at the foot end places one arm next to the first helper's lower arm and her second under the legs below the knees.

The helpers then begin to "bounce" the handicapped person and, using the buoyancy of the water, gradually raise him out of the water. On the fourth "bounce", the helpers make their big effort and lift the handicapped person out of the water. They place their hands on to the edge of the pool and roll the handicapped person off their arms and on to dry land where he is received by other helpers (Fig. 81).

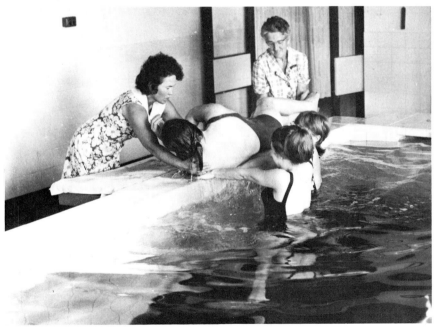

Fig. 81.   *Rolling the handicapped person out of the pool*

Chapter 8

HANDLING HANDICAPPED RIDERS

S. Y. Saywell, F.C.S.P.

Following all the instructions in Chapters 3 and 4, handling severely disabled riders requires few adaptations. From the basic principles, most helpers will have gained insight into the types of disability they may be required to assist. Practical demonstrations may be given by the group physiotherapist whenever new helpers enrol with the riding group.

During a brief assessment period, clothing should be noted and all buttons and/or laces fastened. Wheelchair seat-belts must be released and an explanation of the method of transfer from chair to pony is given. The transfer may be through the standing position using one or two helpers, in which case the handicapped person must turn to face the horse or with his back to it.

Assistance may then be needed to climb one, two or three steps of a mounting block. A third person may be needed here to place the feet in the proper position. The mount may then be concluded as follows, using two helpers:

1. Both legs forward across the saddle, then turning the rider, taking one leg over the horse's neck to assume the correct position.
2. Sitting the rider on the saddle facing sideways towards the person lifting, turning to face the horse's ears, taking the appropriate leg over the horse's neck.
3. Sitting the rider in the normal position, allowing the legs to separate to appropriate sides.

The Severely Handicapped Heavyweight

This type of rider poses the most difficult problems in mounting. He may be a heavyweight teenager with muscular dystrophy or spina bifida, or an adult with, for example, disseminated sclerosis, para-plegia or hemiplegia (perhaps the most difficult of all to handle owing to the gross lack of balance).

It is important that the mounting block or ramp is high enough to allow the rider to remain standing at the level he would put his foot into the stirrup.

The Totally Dependent Rider

The lightweight rider can be lifted bodily from chair to saddle, with one or two helpers as necessary (Fig. 82).

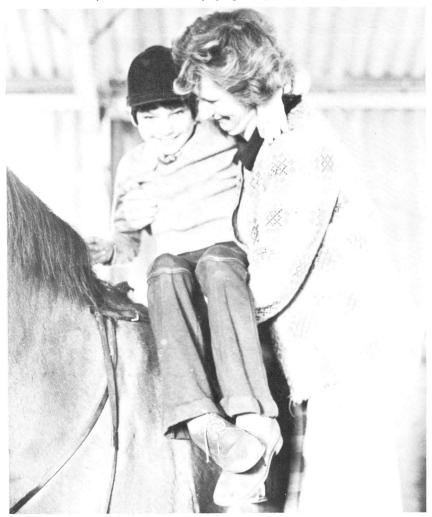

Fig. 82. *The lightweight rider presents no problem*

The heavyweight may require a mechanical lift. Such a hoist, mounted on a gantry, must be high enough to clear the saddle. Ponies and helpers must be well trained to the hoist before introducing the handicapped rider. A team leader should be chosen who is responsible for commanding the movements. Slings are adjusted round the rider's seat and trunk or an adapted transit chair with appropriate attachments used. This will give greater support to the rider and prevent his seat from slipping between the slings. If able to do so, the rider may then wind himself to the required height in order to clear his seat before lowering into the saddle. Helpers guide the rider, taking the legs each side of the pony's neck, and when necessary operate the hoist.

Further adjustments are made quietly a few paces away from the hoist area, one person being responsible for fixing the hoist in the rest position.

Note: All hoists must be inspected and conform to the requirements of the Inspector of Weights and Measures. Annual inspection is required for insurance purposes. Weekly or monthly maintenance, according to use, is essential.

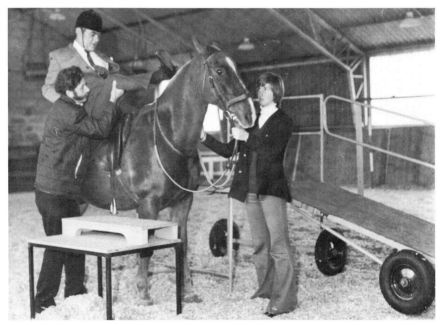

Fig. 83.   *Taking the appropriate leg over the horse's neck*

Ramps

Specially designed ramps are to be found at centres specialising in handling numbers of handicapped riders. These may be built as fixtures when land can be spared for such a purpose, an example of which can be seen at Chigwell, Essex.

The mobile mounting ramp, designed by Miss J. Pringle, M.C.S.P., planned by Wynn Jones Andrews and Associates, of 22 High Street, Haverfordwest, Pembrokeshire, and manufactured by H. J. James and K. J. Edwards of Haverfordwest, is shown in the background of Fig. 83. Such a ramp can be handled in sections by lightweight helpers.

Mounting Blocks

Mounting blocks on the principle of nests of tables as shown in Fig. 83 are easy for the helpers to handle and are stable for the rider. The rider's foot must be on a level with his normal stirrup length when he is on top of the block.

USEFUL ADDRESSES

Organisations

Action for the Crippled Child, Vincent House, Springfield Road, Horsham, Sussex. *Helps all handicapped children, particularly through research.*

Association for Spina Bifida and Hydrocephalus, 30 Devonshire Street, London W1N 2EB. *Supports and helps patients and families and promotes and sponsors research.*

British Council for Rehabilitation of the Disabled, Tavistock House (South), Tavistock Square, London WC1H 9LB. *Arranges courses and conferences with special reference to employment, disseminates information and runs an engineering department concerned with aids to mobility.*

British Polio Fellowship, Bell Close, West End Road, Ruislip, Middlesex. *Fosters fellowship between victims and provides a personal welfare service.*

Central Council for the Disabled, 34 Eccleston Square, London SW1V 1PE. *Deals with all aspects of disablement.*

Disabled Drivers' Association, Ashwellthorpe Hall, Ashwellthorpe, Norwich, Norfolk NOR 89W. *Gives personal advice and guidance and maintains contact with Government departments and local authorities.*

Disabled Living Foundation, 346 Kensington High Street, London W14 8NS. *Runs an information and advice centre and an exhibition of aids and books.*

Disablement Income Group, Toynbee Hall, 28 Commercial Street, London E1. *Works for economic and social improvements for the disabled.*

Invalid Children's Aid Association, 126 Buckingham Palace Road, London SW1W 9SB. *Supports and helps families with a chronic sick or handicapped child.*

Kids, 17 Sedlescome Road, London SW6 1RE. *Provides holidays for socially and physically handicapped children.*

The Lady Hoare Trust for Thalidomide and Other Physically Handicapped Children, 7 North Street, Midhurst, West Sussex. *Helps financially and in rehabilitation and with technical innovations.*

Multiple Sclerosis Society, 4 Tachbrook Street, London SW1V 1SJ. *Encourages research and helps sufferers.*

National Children's Bureau, 8 Wakley Street, London EC1V 7QE. *Conducts research and publishes results and other literature and films; organises conferences and groups.*

National Society for Mentally Handicapped Children, Pembridge Hall, 17 Pembridge Square, London W2 4EP. *Organises residential centres, physiotherapy, a bookshop and courses.*

Possum Users Association, Kerridge, 25 World's End Lane, Weston Turville, Aylesbury, Buckinghamshire. *Helps sufferers and raises funds.*

Queen Elizabeth's Foundation for the Disabled, Leatherhead, Surrey. *Responsible for four adult residential units offering training and employment, and convalescence and holidays.*

Riding for the Disabled Association, National Equestrian Centre, Kenilworth, Warwickshire CV8 2LR. *Provides facilities for all disabled people wishing to ride who have medical approval.*

Spastics Society, 12 Park Crescent, London W1N 4EQ. *Runs schools, residential and day care centres, hostels and training establishments.*

Spinal Injuries Association, 24 Nutford Place, London W1H 6AN. *Provides information for the benefit of paraplegics and tetraplegics, promotes research, and arranges conferences, courses and exhibitions.*

Suppliers of hoists
S. Burvill & Son, 39 Primrose Road, Walton-on-Thames, Surrey. *Burvill hydraulic car hoist.*

Gimson & Co. Ltd., Vulcan Road, Leicester LE5 3EA. *Gimson stairlifts.*

Highfield Engineering & Design Bromsgrove Ltd., 109–111 Speedwell Road, Hay Mills, Birmingham B25 8HW. *Spa bath lift.*

Mecanaids Ltd., St. Catherine Street, Gloucester GL1 2BX. *Mecalift and Autolift.*

F. J. Payne & Son Ltd., Mill Street, Osney, Oxford. *New Oxford Hoist.*

Railvalift Ltd., 73 Park Avenue, Potters Bar, Hertfordshire. *Railvalift harness.*

Surgical Medical Laboratories, 12 Hutton Grove, Finchley, London N12. *Major track and transportable hoists.*

Wessex Medical Equipment Co., 108 The Hundred, Romsey, Hampshire. *Wessex electric hoist.*

Zimmer (G.B.) Ltd., 134 Brompton Road, London SW3 1JB. *Heavy-duty patient lifter.*

Suppliers of beds
Egerton Hospital Equipment Ltd., Tower Hill, Horsham, Sussex RH13 7JT. *Tilting and turning bed. Stand-up bed.*

J. Nesbit-Evans & Co. Ltd., Wednesbury, Staffordshire WS10 7BL. *King's Fund bed.*

Tutor Holdings Ltd., 17 Market Place, Henley-on-Thames, Oxfordshire RG9 1LT. *Electrically operated bed.*

Western Waterbed, 281 Finchley Road, London NW3. *Domestic and hospital waterbeds.*

Suppliers of wheelchairs
Amesbury Surgical Appliances Ltd., South Mill Road, Amesbury, Salisbury, Wiltshire. *Children's chairs, both powered and non-powered.*

Andrews MacLaren Ltd., Station Works, Long Buckby, Northampton NN6 7PF. *Folding pushchairs in junior sizes.*

W. and F. Barrett Ltd., Emery Road, Brislington Trading Estate, Bristol BS4 5PH. *Non-powered chairs, adult and junior.*

Bentley of Birmingham, 21 Shakespeare Street, Sparkhill, Birmingham B11. *Bencraft non-powered chairs, adult and junior.*

Biddle Engineering Co. Ltd., 103 Stourbridge Road, Halesowen, West Midlands B63 3UB. *Powered indoor and outdoor chairs with 14 in., 16 in. and 17 in. seat width.*

Braune of Stroud (Batric), Griffin Mill, Thrupp, Stroud, Gloucestershire. *Powered outdoor chairs.*

Everest & Jennings Ltd., Zimmer House, 134 Brompton Road, London SW3. *Powered and non-powered chairs in child, junior and adult sizes.*

Modern Tubular Productions Ltd., 188 High Street, Egham, Surrey. *Non-powered chairs, adult and junior.*

Tan Sad Allwin Ltd., Toll End Road, Great Bridge, Tipton, Staffordshire. *Non-powered and power conversion chairs, adult and junior.*

Travelectrix (Jersey) Ltd., Route de la Haule, St. Brelaide, Jersey, Channel Islands. *Traveller battery-operated electric outdoor wheelchairs.*

Vessa Ltd., Paper Mill Lane, Alton, Hampshire. *Non-powered chairs, adult and junior.*

ADVERTISEMENT SECTION

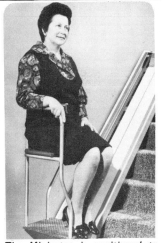
Index to advertisers

FOLDING PUSHCHAIRS
for the HANDICAPPED YOUNG
Buggy Major

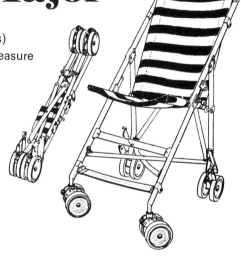

Weighs only **5.4** kg (12 lbs)

Carries up to **59** kg (126 lbs)

Folds easily and quickly to measure only 107 × 19 × 16.5 cm. (42″ × 7½″ × 6½″).

- All wheels well sprung
- Front wheels fully castoring
- Brake on both sides at rear
- Adjustable footrest
- Easy to steer
- Easy to carry
- Easily transported in car, bus, train or airliner

SEPARATE SEAT ATTACHMENT

A separate fabric seat attachment with sides and two lap straps, is available for children needing extra support. The fabric slips quickly and safely over existing seat and framework.

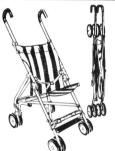

Baby Buggy

WEIGHS ONLY **2.7** kg (6 lbs)

INVALID MODEL FOR YOUNG CHILDREN
aged 6 months to 3 years

Folds simply to measure only 103 × 16.4 × 16.4 cm (41″ × 6½″ × 6½″)

- Ankle and lap straps
- Well sprung wheels
- Made from polished aluminium
- Safety brake
- Can be carried over the arm

ANDREWS MACLAREN LTD
Station Works, Long Buckby, Northampton, England NN6 7PF
Telephone: *Long Buckby 842662*

122

Scandia Toilet Aid

Sturdy and portable, this toilet aid is ideal for those who have difficulty in sitting down or getting up.

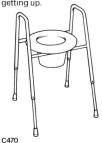

C470

C455

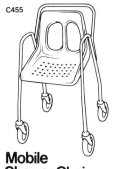

Mobile Shower Chair

Designed for maximum security and convenience – the arms and back provide firm support for the patient.

Adjustable Raised Toilet Seat

Easy to install and remove. Adjusts up to 7" above normal height.

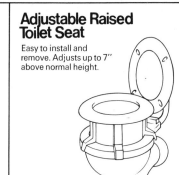

C466

Polypropylene Raised Toilet Seat

Designed to fit all standard toilets – comfortable, lightweight and easy to clean.

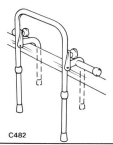

C457

Swedish Bath Grip

Made in chromium-plated steel tubing it is adjusted to the thickness of the bath by two handwheels.

C482

C412

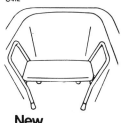

New Simplex Bath Seat

An absolute must for all those who have difficulty getting in and out of the bath – will easily adjust to fit most bath widths.

For years Carters have been dedicated to making the bathroom a safer place for convalescent, disabled and geriatric patients. This range of aids is designed with the thought and care, based on a hundred years of Carters experience. They are comfortable, easy to use and clean and are designed to blend with the bathroom setting. Carters make many more aids to make bathrooms safer. For full details fill in the coupon.

CARTERS
CARTERS (J&A) Ltd
PUT SAFETY FIRST
IN THE BATHROOM

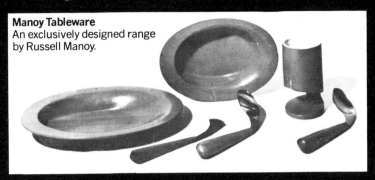
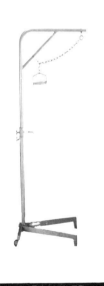
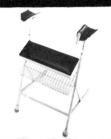
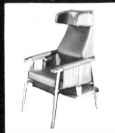
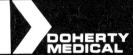
125

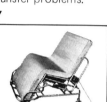
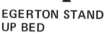
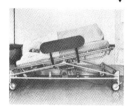
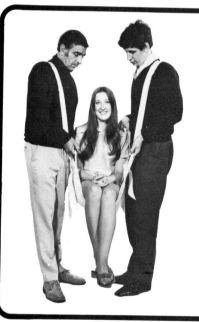

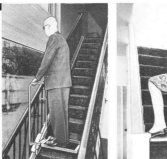

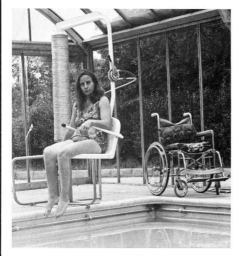

The SPA Pool Lift (left) enables the handicapped with swimming capability to use a swimming pool without assistance, leaving and returning to a wheelchair safely and comfortably.

Patients can be lifted in and out of a Hydrotherapy Pool without effort simply by the movement of a small control lever.

The SPA Bath Lift (below) Smooth silent lifting, free from the snatch and swing associated with mobile hoists, ensures that patients are relaxed and free from tension, making bathing easier. Height adjustment at the touch of a lever simplifies both washing and drying.

photograph by courtesy of Baroness Masham

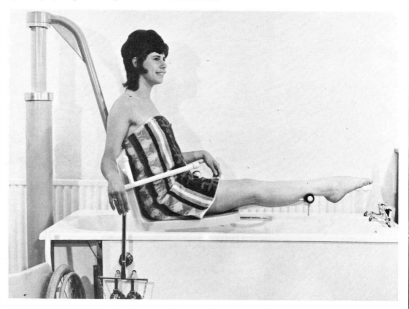

The Droitwich Bathing System combines the Spa Bath Lift and the Droitwich Wheelchair providing 'bed to bath' facility. The patient is lifted direct from and returned to the wheelchair.

HIGHFIELD ENGINEERING AND DESIGN (BROMSGROVE) LTD.
109/111 SPEEDWELL ROAD, BIRMINGHAM, B25 8HW
Tel. 021-772-4845

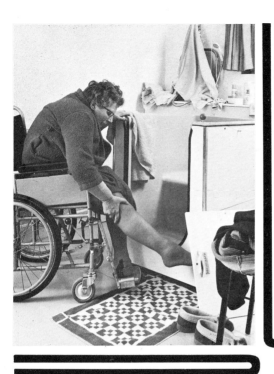
129

travel in comfort
for home, garden, town & country

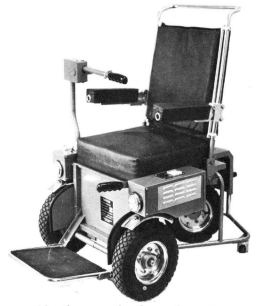

ultra~lightweight single lever occupant controlled battery~powered wheelchair

14 mile range at $3\frac{1}{2}$ m.p.h.
built~in battery charger
automatic magnetic brake

Just a few of the features built into the 100S series wheelchair

For more details write to
TRAVELECTRIX (JERSEY) LIMITED
Route de la Haule, JERSEY, Channel Islands
or ring Vera Campbell, Southwold 2087

How to turn Nurse Mary Jones into a champion weight lifter.

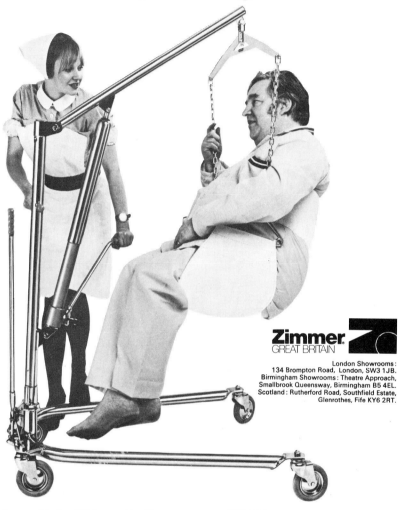

Zimmer
GREAT BRITAIN

Nurse Mary Jones weighs just 106 lb. yet with a Zimmer Heavy Duty Patient Lifter she can lift a 280 lb. patient with just one hand. The powerful hydraulic pump simply removes all the effort.

Zimmer, always striving to improve on the best, have incorporated several design innovations. They include a new spreader bar which prevents swinging and makes for even more positive positioning of the patient – and a lower base which is adjustable from 24" to 35", enabling the Lifter to be moved through narrow door openings.

Instant, mobile, patient lifting is available at any hour of the day or night with this sturdy, versatile model, which operates completely independent of power supply.

131

INDEX